Rodolfo Araújo

Oral Care Carried Out by Nursing Teams

Rodolfo Araújo

Oral Care Carried Out by Nursing Teams

The Importance of Oral Care in Intensive Care Units

ScienciaScripts

Imprint

Cover image: www.ingimage.com

This book is a translation from the original published under ISBN 978-3-330-99745-5.

Publisher:
Sciencia Scripts
is a trademark of
Dodo Books Indian Ocean Ltd. and OmniScriptum S.R.L publishing group

120 High Road, East Finchley, London, N2 9ED, United Kingdom
Str. Armeneasca 28/1, office 1, Chisinau MD-2012, Republic of Moldova, Europe
Managing Directors: Ieva Konstantinova, Victoria Ursu
info@omniscriptum.com

Printed at: see last page
ISBN: 978-620-8-61494-2

To GOD, a constant presence in my life, allowing me to fulfil yet another dream;

To my grandfather, José Gomes de Araújo, an example of life, for all his teachings and the trust he placed in me;

To my PARENTS, Nelson and Ana Araújo, for their dedication, encouragement and support over a lifetime, indispensable for turning my dream into reality;

To my SISTERS, Andreza and Renata, for their words of strength and encouragement;

To my SISTERS, Lucas, Louise and Rafael, for being part of my life and for the countless joys and smiles they brought me;

To my WIFE, Amanda, for her constant affection, companionship and love, even in times of discouragement;

To my CHILD, Sophia, an inexhaustible source of love and dedication, for coming into my life at the right time, making me a new man.

ACKNOWLEDGEMENTS

To my supervisor Prof Dr Adriano Maia Corrêa, for his attention and collaboration during this achievement;

To those responsible for the management and administration of the institutions we visited, for allowing us in and making our study possible;

To the professionals from the nursing teams interviewed, for their willingness to participate in our research;

To Prof Dr[1] Regina Madruga Tavares, for her attention and collaboration in the statistical analysis of the research;

To the Pará Regional Nursing Council (COREN), for providing the information required for this research;

To all the colleagues in the 2006/2008 master's programme, for the rewarding interaction and the valuable information and knowledge exchanged over the course of these two years;

To all those who, whether with words or attitudes, helped make this study a success.

"Wisdom is not given to us; we have to discover it for ourselves after a journey that no one can spare us or make for us."

(Marcel Proust)

SUMMARY

In an attempt to establish a profile of the perception and performance of oral health care provided to patients in intensive care units by nursing teams, a study was carried out with 402 interviews guided by a questionnaire. The study population was made up of nursing professionals divided into three training categories: nurses, nursing technicians and nursing assistants who work in public and private hospital institutions providing services in intensive care units in the city of Belém-PA. Dentistry has developed significantly in this area, linking scientific discoveries and practical applications in the field of prevention and restoring oral health. This reflection correlates with the research carried out in this study, which returned results suggesting that oral hygiene care provided to patients hospitalised in ICUs is scarce and inadequate, and that changes are needed to the care currently provided, especially in the nursing team's nosocomial environment. The presence of a dental surgeon, the dissemination of preventive dentistry knowledge and the use of specific oral hygiene resources are measures suggested as attempts to solve the difficulties presented in maintaining oral health and treating oral diseases, which affect the general health of hospitalised patients. Interdisciplinary action in the care of these individuals is advocated in order to achieve a better quality of life by preventing or minimising the oral pathologies present.
KEY WORDS: 1. hospital dentistry. 2. interdisciplinarity. 3. oral health 4. oral care.

SUMMARY

CHAPTER 1

INTRODUCTION

In Brazil, dentistry and medicine are separate professions and the treatment of oral problems is the responsibility of the dental surgeon. However, the patient cannot be divided into areas; the evolution of health concepts has been converging towards a vision of man as an integrated whole, a biopsychosocial being. In the field of dentistry, there has historically been a concentration on individual clinical care, in consulting rooms, isolated from the community and other professions. In line with this reality, there is a greater need for specialised dental training to care for hospitalised patients. In general, patients in hospitals or clinics for long periods of time do not receive proper oral health care, which should be provided regularly.

Oral prevention needs to be implemented to avoid the loss of teeth and its consequences for systemic health. Therefore, preventive care of the oral cavity in a hospital environment should include periodic examination, inspecting for changes in the normal aspects of these tissues, and referral to curative care whenever lesions or pain are noticed. Also necessary are: proper tooth brushing, flossing, care of dentures and ensuring that they are properly fitted, and instruction in the use of other instruments that prevent infections of the oral mucosa.

Intensive care units (ICUs) arose from the need to improve and concentrate material and human resources for the care of critically ill patients who were still considered recoverable, and the need for constant observation, continuous medical and nursing care, centralising patients in a specialised unit.

The ICU patient needs excellent care, directed not only at the pathophysiological problems, but also at the psychosocial, environmental and family issues that become closely intertwined with the physical illness. The essence of multidisciplinarity in intensive care is not in the environments or special equipment, but in the decision-making process, based on a solid understanding of the patient's physiological and psychological conditions and new therapies. The patient's sense of comfort should also be taken into account. HALLET (1984) emphasised that, according to the opinion of the patients who were analysed, a sanitised oral cavity provided a feeling of well-being. In addition to the unpleasant odour associated with halitosis, there is the social aspect of not having a clean mouth.

It is essential that ICU patients receive sufficient oral care during their hospitalisation in order to prevent the onset of oral pathologies and possible complications of existing oral diseases.

In very ill patients, bacteria present in the oral cavity, which are predominantly gram-positive, can change to gram-negative anaerobic characteristics, since microorganisms that colonise the oral cavity of these patients are virulent compared to naturally occurring organisms, consequently the risk of infection is high, providing unsatisfactory responses to bacterial invasion of the lungs (JENKINS, 1989). Pathogens commonly responsible for nosocomial pneumonia are found colonising dental plaque and the oral mucosa of these patients. However, good oral hygiene techniques are able to prevent the spread of infection from the oral cavity to the respiratory tract.

Many studies have documented that patients admitted to intensive care units have poorer oral hygiene than non-hospitalised patients and have a higher prevalence of colonisation of respiratory pathogens on their teeth and oral mucosa. The lack of adequate oral hygiene in these patients optimises the conditions for bacterial growth. The increased volume and complexity of dental plaque can promote bacterial interactions between native plaque bacteria and respiratory pathogens, contributing to the development of respiratory diseases such as pneumonia and chronic obstructive pulmonary disease.

Pneumonia is one of the main causes of hospitalisation worldwide. In Brazil, it represents the fourth leading cause of hospitalisation in the elderly and is also an important cause of death in these individuals. In the USA, it is estimated that approximately 60,000 deaths from pneumonia occur each year in the elderly (Ministry of Health, 2001).

While healthcare teams remain uncertain about the ideal way to treat their patients, especially in developed countries, society is increasingly concerned about the personal, social and economic costs of current practices in medicine and particularly in intensive care. By maintaining patients' lives through the replacement of organ functions by artificial means, the dying process is being lengthened, often generating suffering for family members and patients, without any concern for the patient's health.

The aim is to improve survival or quality of life. However, promoting quality of life in an intensive care environment becomes a difficult issue, because at such a critical moment the overriding concern is the fight against death, using all the invasive invasive procedures.

The defence mechanisms from the upper airways (UA) to the tracheobronchial tree include hair, highly vascularised mucous membranes with ciliated epithelium and a mucous mantle that traps inhaled particles and is transported to the oropharynx by the ciliated epithelium. Endotracheal intubation is one of the procedures that reduces the effectiveness of nasal and pulmonary defences (SAFAR and CAROLINE, 1982). It is therefore consistent to state that critically ill intubated patients have a particularly high risk of developing an infection such as nosocomial pneumonia.

As the available literature and discussions with various members of the Nursing Teams who were approached during the period of the study in question revealed a great diversity in dental interventions, many of them without adequate scientific support, we propose to indicate possible mouth hygiene protocols and subsequent controls for various clinical situations common to individuals affected by pneumonia, particularly as it is one of the most common diseases in the older age group of the population, especially when they are bed-bound.

CHAPTER 2

LITERATURE REVIEW

2.1 INTEGRATION AND INTERDISCIPLINARITY

It is understood that the individual must be understood in all their physical, psychological and social integrity, aiming to improve the quality of life and well-being of the patient, through the integration of health professionals (KOIZUMI and CIANCIARULLO, 1978). This is why we emphasise the importance of preventive measures, since they are less costly and more comprehensive than individual curative and rehabilitative treatments (GLASSMAN et al., 1994). Thus, the aim of primary promotion in dentistry is to prevent the development of diseases or to reverse them in the early stages, such as caries, periodontal diseases and oral cancer.

Men's health care in Brazil's public healthcare network is usually seen as having therapeutic, emergency or palliative objectives, following a secular curative or generalist care model with few professionals who carry out multiple activities with superficial knowledge. However, changes have been noticed and its differentiation can be seen in the multiplicity of professional areas linked to health and the subdivisions into specialities and sub-specialities. This has resulted in knowledge and assistance with greater competence and efficiency, but on the other hand we can see a loss of vision of the individual's integrity. Today, knowledge is spreading faster and is divided into different disciplines. However, there is a need to transcend multifaceted knowledge and integrate analyses. Integrated knowledge is aimed at communication and dialogue, generating a mutual relationship between the concepts of the disciplines, creating new knowledge or seeking solutions to various health problems (CARVALHO FILHO and PAPALÉO NETTO, 2000).

According to Vilela and Mendes (2003), health is considered to be an eminently interdisciplinary area and the integration of disciplines in human resources training courses in this field could certainly lead to the training of professionals who are more committed to the reality of health and its social transformation. The condition of illness generates feelings such as incapacity, dependence, insecurity and a sense of loss of control over oneself. Patients see hospitalisation as a factor of depersonalisation because they recognise the difficulty in maintaining their identity, intimacy and privacy. The hospital environment is stressful for various reasons, essentially for the patient, as they lose control over factors that affect them and on which they depend for their survival. In addition, hospitalisation is distressing because it highlights the fragility to which they are subject, due to emotional and physical exposure.

Each professional performs specific functions within a joint team plan, with co-responsibility in the decision-making process. Thus, the assumptions of this integration have been present in healthcare for some time and, in recent decades, we have noticed the need for transformations in relation to specialised knowledge. There are many difficulties in implementing disciplinary interaction, which requires overcoming historical limits, restructuring the training of human resources and renewing interpersonal relationships between health professionals (REZENDE, 2005).

The value of oral health care in preventing pneumonia is clear. This conclusion was recorded during a literature review on the importance of dental care for patients in intensive care units, carried out by Morais et al (2006). It was found that the monitoring of organs and systems that are not the direct cause of the problem that led to the patient's condition should not be forgotten. This attention prevents the deterioration of another organ or system that could contribute to an unfavourable prognosis of the case. This also includes the stomatognathic system, which should receive due attention. Since the prevalence, extent and severity of periodontal diseases is very high in the population. Poor oral hygiene is a characteristic finding in ICU patients. These authors also stated that, until now, the obstacle often faced by the dental surgeon in joining multidisciplinary teams in the ICU was the low priority given to dental procedures in the face of the numerous problems presented by the patient. However, the literature has clearly and forcefully demonstrated the influence of the oral condition on the evolution of the condition of hospitalised patients. Studies that included this work indicated that ICU patients had poor oral hygiene, with significantly more biofilm than individuals living in society. These patients were also more likely to have their oral biofilm colonised by respiratory pathogens. The amount and complexity of the oral biofilm also increased with the length of hospitalisation. These results suggest that colonisation of the oral biofilm by pathogens, especially respiratory pathogens, may be a specific source of important nosocomial infection in the ICU. Since the bacteria present in the mouth can be aspirated and cause aspiration pneumonia. In view of pathophysiological data showing a possible relationship between dental care and nosocomial pneumonia, the dental surgeon could be added to the multi-professional team for the benefit of critically ill patients. Since poor oral hygiene and the presence of periodontal disease in ICU patients are undoubtedly another factor that can favour the development of nosocomial pneumonia. Firstly, because this oral condition results in a high concentration of pathogens in the saliva that can be aspirated into the lungs in abundance. Secondly, the oral biofilm can harbour pulmonary pathogens and promote their growth. And finally, the periodontal pathogens could facilitate colonisation of the upper airways by lung pathogens.

2.2 HOSPITAL DENTISTRY

Awareness of the contribution that each speciality can make to health care gives biomedical professionals greater responsibilities (Du GAS, 1984). The incorporation of new knowledge and its practical application by professionals who are more committed to social, professional and human responsibilities, who are aware of the implications of oral diseases on systemic health and who are committed to improving the morbidity and well-being of patients, are necessary in order to provide better care for senile individuals.

Brunner and Suddarth (1992) quoted the following: nursing is the assessment and improvement of the state, capacity and health potential of human beings. Still within this same reasoning, the authors point out that the nursing process is used to help patients use their attributes, seeking to achieve and maintain their well-being at the highest possible levels, within their physical and psychosocial limitations.

Loesche et al. (1995), in a study at the University of Michigan correlating oral health with lifestyle and medical status, pointed out that medically healthy people had excellent oral health, while individuals who were ill had several tooth losses or were edentulous.

According to Puricelli and Wells (1996), the speciality of dentistry "Oral and Maxillofacial Surgery and Traumatology (OMFT)" enables other specialities to practice in hospitals, adding dentistry to the multidisciplinary activities in the health area. Among the difficulties experienced by CTBMF professionals, there is a lack of clarification from nursing and medical staff on how to properly refer a patient to an oral and maxillofacial dentist, and in many cases medical corporatism ends up favouring doctors who are not trained in oral and maxillofacial treatment. The authors advocate the creation of new disciplines to keep up with future health trends, highlighting the need to integrate dentistry with veterinary medicine, intrauterine treatments, space research, specialised software, robotics, bioengineering and geriatrics. It was concluded that dentistry could be integrated into the care of hospital patients with oral health problems or whose condition is aggravated by the association of these problems, such as those with syndromes, oral invalids or coma patients, as well as expanding the field of teaching and practice of dentistry, for prevention, research and care.

Orientation should be extended to all the different segments of the interdisciplinary team, as this practice, which is fundamental in preventive dentistry, prevents contact with dental professionals from occurring too late. Patients, family members, doctors, nursing staff, carers and other members of the team involved need to be made aware of patients' potential dental problems and the importance of regular oral hygiene, especially if debilitating systemic conditions worsen (IACOPINO, 1997; REYNOLDS, 1997). Local and systemic complications can arise from maintaining poor oral health in these patients.

Erickson (1997) concluded that foods such as chewing gums and sugar-free candies with effects on the remaining salivary function can be indicated, as well as fluoride and antibacterial agents that reduce the risks associated with xerostomia. In hospitals, nurses are responsible for oral hygiene, among other things. The dentist's guidance is therefore necessary for the procedures to be carried out correctly. For this reason, hygiene programmes should be designed taking into account individual needs.

Developments in dental science and practice in recent times have brought recognition, such as the first Oral Health Report from the US Department of Oral Health, which officially states that oral health is an integral part of general health. This has led to the need for greater action, giving greater commitment to research that translates scientific evidence into dental practice, as well as real benefits for people with oral problems (GENCO & GROSSI, 1998).

Malnutrition is another factor responsible for high morbidity rates, slow wound healing, increased hospital infection rates, longer hospital stays, especially in ICUs, and higher re-hospitalisation rates, as well as high costs for the health system. Medical and nursing courses currently give little importance to patients' nutritional status, which is directly related to the patient's clinical evolution. In this case, the lack of knowledge on the subject makes it difficult to recognise and correct a given clinical-hospital situation (WAITZBERG et al., 1998).

In order to reduce the effects of xerostomia, salivary substitutes can be used, which improve the moisture and texture of the tongue and mucous membranes (POTTER and PERRY, 1999), stimulate salivation and alleviate the effects of dry mouth. Unconscious individuals are susceptible to dry, mucous-thickened secretions due to their inability to eat, mouth breathing or oxygen therapy, as well as not swallowing the salivary secretions that accumulate in the oral cavity. Salivary secretions contain bacteria, mainly gram-negative, which cause pneumonia if they are aspirated and reach the lungs. These patients must be protected from aspiration and suffocation and require special oral care. Dentists and the healthcare team must work in an integrated manner for patients who present physiological and pathological alterations with manifestations in the oral cavity (SOUZA et al., 2001).

The authors also refer to the oral alterations commonly found and described in the leaflets of these medications, which are characterised by a decrease in salivary flow, leading to a greater number of caries lesions and periodontal disease, canker sores, mucositis, dysplasia, speech difficulties, candidiasis, dentin sensitivity, glossitis, lichenoid reactions, erythema, halitosis, among others.

Timby (2001) classifies patients into three levels: independent, partially dependent and totally dependent, with the highest incidence of independent and partially dependent patients. This classification in terms of degree of dependence helps with excellent planning of nursing care, sizing of human and material resources, planning of nursing care, forecasting of care costs and better distribution of activities between members of the nursing team. Independent patients are those who are conscious and capable and can perform their own oral hygiene using the bathroom sink. For these patients, the oral care carried out by the nursing team is varied and, even if conscious patients can carry out their own oral hygiene, it is the professional's responsibility to encourage them to do so and to check that appropriate techniques are being carried out. When caring for partially or totally dependent patients, the nurse may need to brush the teeth of many bedridden patients and will need to be familiar with appropriate techniques such as flossing.

In addition to the routine oral hygiene materials and instruments, these patients will need an emesis tank.

The author also states that bedridden patients have the resources for oral hygiene provided by the nursing staff. The use of toothpaste, soft brushes and dental floss is recommended. However, patients with a higher level of dependency or with oral pathologies need more assistance with hygiene.

Knowing that saliva has a lubricating, moisturising and antibiotic function, one of the most common reactions in the oral cavity seen in hospitalised patients is xerostomia, which is characterised by the subjective sensation of dry mouth and is caused by a decrease in salivary flow, which can influence nutrient intake. Patients who need special hospital care, in particular, may have difficulty chewing and swallowing and therefore tend to avoid certain types of food, especially those with a crunchy, dry and sticky consistency (HARRIS, 2002).

Nursing has developed a lot in the caring process, and is seen as the art and science of caring. Caring has become much more than an act, it is an attitude of occupation, concern, responsibility and involvement, as well as involving affection, which demands commitment from professional nurses towards their fellow human beings. Nursing can't, and shouldn't, focus only on the illness, but on the individual as a whole, who, because they are ill, needs personal and special care (PUPULIM and SAWADA, 2002).

A poor lifestyle leads to malnutrition, which in turn leads to greater morbidity and mortality. Indications of poor nutritional status are: illness, poor eating habits, tooth loss or toothache, economic hardship, use of multiple medications, involuntary weight loss or gain, need for help with self-care. Interventions to treat nutritional problems include social services, oral health, mental health, medication use, nutritional education and support (HARRIS, 2002).

Chewing is one of the guarantees of the absorption of nutrients that are fundamental to life. The dentist's role in the patient's overall care is to analyse, intervene and control the patients' functional oral conditions, contributing to their speedy recovery and return to normal life, away from hospital beds (BRUNETTI & MONTENEGRO, 2003). From this point of view, malnutrition can occur in 19 to 80% of hospitalised patients, due to various morbid states and after hospital admission. Up to 70% of initially malnourished patients suffer a gradual worsening of their nutritional status during hospitalisation. As a result, food intake in hospital falls as a result of reduced capacity to utilise food due to inefficient chewing or loss of appetite. As a result of malnutrition, the patient's general condition and response to treatment are affected. The authors also state that tooth loss and the use of dentures can lead to a reduction in chewing efficiency of around 75 to 85 per cent and, consequently, to less consumption of fresh meat, fruit and vegetables. Food preferences are modified as a result of food consistency. Foods with lower energy value are consumed, as well as diets low in fibre and protein, which influences the patient's nutritional status. Various causes lead to difficulty swallowing in patients, such as poor dentition, Alzheimer's disease (AD) or other dementias, traumatic brain injury, Parkinson's disease, amyotrophic lateral sclerosis, multiple sclerosis, debilitation after heart surgery, recurrent pneumonia, oesophageal reflux or cancer, brain surgery or prolonged intubation. Indications of swallowing difficulties include: a change in voice (wet and gurgling), coughing or choking when eating or drinking, drooling, packing food down, poor lip closure, unintelligible speech and excessively long feeding times. In addition to the medical and nursing team, dentists, speech therapists, nutritionists and physiotherapists, among others, may be needed to treat patients with these symptoms. Enteral or parenteral nutrition can be justified when the patient is unable to swallow or consume adequate calories and nutrients through natural food.

Lack of knowledge of the side effects of medications recommended by doctors on the oral cavity has consequences for patients' health: approximately 45 per cent of the medications prescribed for this population can cause adverse reactions (MONTENEGRO, 2003).

Decreased salivation is often caused by autoimmune diseases, irradiation in head and neck cancer, as well as medication. Also known as xerostomia, it results in various alterations, such as gingivitis, increased tooth decay, halitosis, reduced sense of taste, difficulty chewing, swallowing and speaking. For this reason, treatment for xerostomia must include identifying the causal factor (CASSOLATO and TURNBULL, 2004).

A comparative sample study carried out in Austria and the UK evaluates how age and tooth loss can affect oral health and its effects on quality of life. The researchers realised that the greater the number of teeth, the greater the impact on oral health; a factor that indicates a better quality of life. From this perspective, a balanced diet and the consumption of adequate amounts of nutrients can be altered by the absence of frequent dental care and missing teeth. Patients with few functional teeth or ill-fitting dentures have a lower intake of nutrients compared to patients with teeth or adequate replacement of tooth loss. Thus, it was observed that dental issues can increase the risk of mortality. It can be concluded that preventive dental care, aimed at preserving natural teeth and adjusting dentures, reduces the nutritional risk in patients undergoing hospital treatment (STEELE et al., 2004).

The interaction between health professionals and their patients creates a communication channel that will lead to the choice of the best necessary procedure, concluded Basílio et al (2004) when they assessed patients with infective endocarditis, a heart disease with a high morbidity rate that is fatal when not diagnosed and treated in time. Its aetiopathogenesis consists of a combination of bacteremia and other factors, such as heart lesions, which can be congenital and/or acquired, a weakened immune system and/or poor oral hygiene. This pathology can be combated or prevented by reducing the intensity and duration of bacteraemia. According to the authors, the dentist plays a fundamental role at this point in the patient's treatment, combining medical and dental aspects, as antibiotic prophylaxis alone is not considered sufficient to combat this illness. Patients with poor oral health, root abscesses and gingivitis offer the perfect entry point for microorganisms into the bloodstream. Oral prophylaxis techniques can be carried out or guided by dentists in patients with endocarditis, an essential procedure for their recovery or prevention.

Nursing should particularly assess the patient's degree of independence in terms of their ability to fulfil their hygiene needs. This should not be seen as a way of relieving nursing duties, as hygiene care should be encouraged, as should the patient's independence (LAUS and ANSELMI, 2004).

Several statistical studies correlate poor oral health with systemic diseases. We can see that various components of the oral microbiota can cause systemic illnesses, whether they are pathogens capable of promoting lesions in other human tissues, or those responsible for colonisation of the oral biofilm by opportunistic bacteria. Health promotion in specific groups aims to minimise these problems (NASCIMENTO et al., 2005). Therefore, it is of fundamental importance for dentists to be aware of the systemic and oral alterations that a patient requiring hospital care may present (MARTINS FILHO and SANTOS, 2005).

In a study carried out at the Hospital de Caridade e Beneficência de Cachoeira do Sul, Doro et al. (2006) assessed the oral health conditions of hospitalised patients and the conditions that the institution had in place to properly promote oral hygiene for its patients. Undergraduate dentistry students carried out oral examinations and gave oral hygiene instructions to patients and carers. Oral hygiene instructions were also given to nurses and nursing technicians in order to improve the quality of the services provided. It was found that the majority of patients had poor oral health control; many in-patients had prostheses with poor hygiene due to a deficiency on the part of the in-patient, a lack of motivation on the part of carers, a lack of oral hygiene materials and the poor structure of the hospital. The appearance of candidiasis was attributed to the lack of hygiene of the dentures. According to the authors, plaque control is very important for patients in hospital, especially those with systemic illnesses. The use of chlorhexidine has been recommended to prevent periodontal disease when, for some reason, mechanical plaque removal cannot be carried out. Therefore, the hospital lacked dental services, especially to prevent and control oral diseases.

2.3 BIOFILM FORMATION

Dental plaque or dental biofilm are the terms used universally to describe the association of bacteria with the dental surface. Dental plaque was described by Dawes et al. (1973) as a mass that is not eliminated by rinsing with water or air or by chewing, but is soft and adherent and deposited continuously on the tooth surface.

According to Carranza (1992), the oral cavity has one of the most varied microbial populations, with the dorsum of the tongue, the gingival sulcus and dental plaque being the areas of greatest concentration. The mouth has characteristics that facilitate the development of microbial flora, including fungi, bacteria, viruses and protozoa. The temperature of approximately 35° to 37°C, the moisture and nutrients provided by the gingival fluid, epithelial cells and other degradation processes, salivary components and extrinsic nutrients from the diet favour the growth of these microorganisms. Oxygen tension and pH also allow many aerobic bacteria to expand.

Loesche (1993), in his study of swabs from the mouth, proved the presence of filamentous forms facultative anaerobes, spirochetes, Neisseria, facultative Streptococci, Bacterioides, Fusobacterium and Leptotrichia. Microorganisms of the type Staphylococcus, Streptococcus pneumoniae, Klebsiella pneumoniae, Haemoplilus influenzae, Escherichia coli and Franciella tularensis have been found isolated in the mouth in hospital infections.

Biofilm is formed through two distinct phases. In the first phase, negatively charged bacteria can reach a negatively charged surface using their kinetic energy. The second phase is characterised by the accumulation of bacteria by coaggregation with the same species or with other species through mechanisms and structures such as adhesins, pili, glycocalyx, as well as the production of an extracellular polysaccharide matrix (JORGE, 1998).

Leite et al. (1999) observed that the formation of biofilm guarantees bacterial colonies some advantages such as: better communication between cells due to the solution of continuity between them, thus facilitating their biochemical activities, improves the proliferation of bacteria, enables access to niches and resources that could not be reached by isolated cells and, above all, favours defence against antagonistic factors.

The term dental biofilm is used to designate communities of microorganisms (bacteria and/or fungi) adhered to the dental surface and under the continuous action of a flow. It can also be defined as a structured, non-calcified aggregate of microorganisms, adhered to the dental surface, contained in an organic matrix made up of bacterial polymers and substances from the host's saliva and diet (SIMIONATO, 2006).

The initial colonisation phase of biofilm bacteria lasts from 0 to 8 hours, and the bacteria's binding mechanisms predominate, including Van der Waals attractive forces and hydrophobic interactions. Participating in this phase are the microorganisms S. sanguinis, Actinomyces viscous, A. naeslundii and S. mutans. In this same phase, the mechanisms of bacterial adherence to the acquired film and the participation of adhesins and receptors are highlighted. Among the pioneering microorganisms in this process are Streptococcus and Actinomyces. The rapid growth phase lasts from 4 to 48 hours and interbacterial adhesion mechanisms predominate. Participating in this phase are the following bacteria: S. mutans and A. naelundii, S. sanguinis, S. oralis, Fusobacterium nucleatum, S. gordonii, S. oralis, Porphyromonas gingivalis, Prevotella loesheii, A. israelli, C. gingivalis and A. israelii. The remodelling phase begins after 48 hours and continues indefinitely. The total number of microorganisms remains constant, but the microbial composition is more complex (SIMIONATO, 2006).

2.4 METHODS USED TO REDUCE THE RATE OF DENTAL BIOFILM IN HOSPITALISED PATIENTS

Some studies have investigated the role of inadequate oral hygiene in the onset of respiratory infections in patients who have received a certain type of artificial respiration (BAGRAMIAN and HELLER, 1977).

Several studies have documented that hospitalised individuals tend to have poor oral hygiene compared to outpatients and controls in society. This lack of attention to oral hygiene results in an increase in the quantity and complexity of dental plaque, which can favour the interaction of indigenous plaque bacteria with known respiratory pathogens such as Pseudomas aeruginosa and enteric bacilli (KOMIYAMA et al., 1985).

Due to the findings of various studies into the role of bacteria that colonise the oropharynx in the pathogenesis of bacterial pneumonia, some proposals have been made to try to reduce the bacterial load in the oropharynx. Digestive selective decontamination (DSD) is based on the topical application of antibiotics to the surfaces of the gastrointestinal tract, including the oral cavity, in an attempt to reduce the amount of bacteria that could be released and reach the lower respiratory tract and cause a respiratory infection (KERVER et al., 1988; STOUTENBEEK et al., 1987).

After a study on oral hygiene in hospitals, it was concluded that care should be taken when combining chlorhexidine with dentifrices and fluoride, as sodium lauryl sulphate, one of the most commonly used synthetic detergents in dentifrices, is incompatible with chlorhexidine in aqueous solutions, as it reduces its antimicrobial effect (BARKVOLL et al., 1988).

DSD can be carried out using tablets containing polymyxin B, tobramycin and amphotericin B, which have the ability to reduce the colonisation of gram-negative bacilli (SPIJKERVET et al., 1991). However, despite being able to reduce the colonisation of pathogenic bacteria in hospitals, the DSD method does not seem to have an effect on the mortality rate and may favour the selection of bacteria resistant to the antibiotics used in DSD (GASTINNE et al., 1992). Scannapieco et al. (1992) carried out a study assessing the prevalence of respiratory pathogens colonising the mouth in a group of ICU patients, with special attention to dental plaque and mucosa. She found that 65 per cent of the patients examined had respiratory pathogens in their plaque and oral mucosa, including Staphylococcus aureus, Pseudomonas aeruginosa and 10 genera of gram-negative bacilli. These patients had poor oral hygiene, which may, according to the author, influence the colonisation of the oropharynx by respiratory microorganisms and there is also the hypothesis that the normal flora of the mouth harbours some enzymes that alter the surface of the mucosa, making it more favourable for these pathogens to adhere.

Pugin et al. (1991) tested the topical application of antibiotics to the oropharynx as a means of reducing the incidence of ventilator-associated pneumonia and found that the group of patients who received topical application of antibiotics had a reduced rate of respiratory infection compared to patients who did not receive this care. Clarck and Guest (1994) also stated that a daily rinse with chlorhexidine would be enough to maintain low levels of microorganisms in the oral cavity, while Pearson (1996) maintains that toothbrushes are more effective at removing dental plaque than foam swabs.

Another method used is the topical application of oral antiseptics. Chlorhexidine seems to be the agent that comes closest to being ideal for controlling dental biofilm as it has a broad spectrum of action, acting on gram-positive and gram-negative, aerobic and anaerobic bacteria and fungi in the oral mucosa, as well as reducing the ability of microorganisms to adhere to and colonise dental surfaces (RENTON-HARPER et al., 1996; HILDEBRANDT, 1996),

In their study, Deriso et al. (1996) observed that hospitalised patients who underwent a predetermined oral hygiene protocol in which chlorhexidine was applied topically had a lower rate of respiratory infection compared to patients who received a placebo.

Dental plaque pathogens, such as P. gingivalis, produce enzymes (such as proteases) that alter the surface receptors for adhesins of respiratory pathogens such as H. influenzae, which adheres, colonises and can be aspirated and cause lung infection. Bacteria in the mouth, such as P. gingivalis, produce enzymes that degrade the molecules in saliva that normally form a film over pathogens and prevent them from adhering to the mucosal surface. They also produce enzymes that degrade the saliva film on the mucosal surface, exposing the receptors for adhesins from respiratory pathogens. Saliva cytokines from inflammatory periodontal tissues positively regulate the expression of adhesin receptors on the mucosal surface to promote the colonisation of respiratory pathogens (SCANNAPIECO et al., 1998). Gram-negative bacilli, staphylococci, microorganisms and anaerobic flora contribute significantly to pneumonia in ICU patients.

Biofilm bacteria are resistant to phagocytosis and killing by the host's immune system, as well as to the effect of antimicrobial drugs. They evade natural defences and elimination mechanisms, sustaining continuous growth. They release bacterial components into the oral cavity and ulcerate the sulcus epithelium in response to bacterial enzymes and toxins. This means that oral bacteria enter the general circulation. The biofilm consists of a niche of gram-negative bacteria that have the potential to cause local and systemic infections. These bacteria in the bloodstream activate platelet agglutination, forming clots and thrombosis. They are associated with bacteraemia and activate the inflammatory cascade, forming atheromatous plaques (GENCO & GROSSI, 1998).

According to Lindhe and Karring (1999), a layer of dental plaque can only be detected clinically after 24 hours without cleaning the oral cavity. And the absence or technique of oral hygiene adopted will be closely linked to the number and species of microorganisms found in the mouth.

Cardenosa Cendrero et al. (1999) observed the route of tracheal colonisation in the development of ventilator-associated pneumonia and found that 80 out of 100 patients had colonisation during the first day of endotracheal ventilation. The oral cavity is the first source of pathogenic organisms that cause ventilator-associated pneumonia.

In his study, Stiefel (2000) used tooth brushing as a method of controlling the biofilm index and compared the oral health conditions of eight ICU patients before and after tooth brushing. The author found progress in oral health after brushing, but in this study no microbiological tests were carried out on the dental biofilm and the prevalence of respiratory infections in these patients was not checked.

According to Munro et al. (2002), in a survey of ICU patients, oral hygiene care was prioritised at 53.9 out of 100 points. According to the authors, the aggravating factor is that hospitals don't have an oral hygiene protocol to follow. It is the nurses who determine what oral care should be taken to provide comfort to the patient. Some methods were mentioned by the nurses, such as placing a foam swab in the oral cavity with the hand, rinsing with water or foam. However, it has been shown that care is not associated with a reduction in dental plaque or ventilator-associated pneumonia. The authors noted that some equipment and solutions used by nurses are not recommended, such as bicarbonate and hydrogen peroxide solutions, as they remove debris but can cause minor burns if not diluted correctly. Initially, lemon and glycerine stimulate salivation, but they are acids that cause calcification of the teeth and irritation of the mucous membranes. Prolonged use of these substances causes xerostomia, i.e. reduced salivary flow.

Current care practices in the main ICUs are poorly defined and inconsistent, as they do not include a defined oral care component and focus only on patient comfort, not the removal of microorganisms (SILVA and MORAES, 2005).

Simionato (2006) separated dental plaque into five groups: The first was not associated with disease, with a microbiota made up of 85% gram-positive microorganisms, 75% facultative anaerobes, the majority being gram-positive cocci. More than 75% of the microbiota is made up of sanguinis and gram-negative bacilli, but there are high concentrations of S. mutans and Lactobacillus. They are supragingival plaques that rapidly convert dietary carbohydrates into acids.

In the second group, cariogenic dental plaque has low proportions of S. sanguinis and gram-negative bacilli, but high concentrations of S. mutans and Lactobacillus. These are supragingival plaques that quickly convert carbohydrates from the diet into acids.

The third group is dental plaque associated with gingivitis, with a more complex microbiota, with high proportions of filamentous bacteria, mobile bacilli and spirochetes. Dental plaque associated with chronic periodontitis is the fourth group and has strict anaerobes (90%), gram-negative bacteria (75%) and spirochetes (30%) as the main constituents of the subgingival microbiota, with few cocci and Porphyromonas gingivalis and Treponema spp associated.

In the fifth group, dental plaque is associated with aggressive periodontitis. In its localised form it can be scarce, with the presence of Actinobacillus actinomycetecomitans, isolated in the majority of cases. In its generalised form, multiple species may be involved, such as P. gingivalis, E. corrodens, P. intermédia, Capnocytophaga, A. actinomycetemcomitans, generally associated with systemic involvement.

2.5 INFECTION IN THE INTENSIVE CARE UNIT

According to Segretti (1989), some of the main causes of hospital-acquired infections are urinary catheterisations, tracheal intubation, mechanical ventilation and intravascular catheters, as these are invasive methods.

Treloar and Stechmiller (1995) analysed the care of the oropharynx in 16 ICU patients using mechanical ventilation. Clinical and demographic data were recorded each day of hospitalisation through the collection of microorganisms with swabs, tracheal secretions and oral clinical examinations until the ventilation devices were removed. Seven patients had severe xerostomia; ten lip lesions were identified in nine patients; eight tongue lesions were diagnosed in nine patients; and eight mucosal lesions were recorded in nine patients. 44 per cent of the patients showed radiographic evidence consistent with pneumonia. Gram-negative microorganisms were found in the oropharynx and tracheal secretion simultaneously. Although oral cavity hygiene is considered a highly difficult procedure to perform in intubated patients, it is known that the poor state of the oropharynx can be related to the acquisition of nosocomial organisms and this relationship should be given greater attention. Therefore, systematic and clinical analysis of the oropharynx can prevent the onset and worsening of many infections.

According to David (1998), infection is a frequent manifestation in critically ill patients admitted to the ICU. The patient may have a community-acquired infection, i.e. one that is already present or incubating at the time of hospital admission, or a nosocomial infection, defined as appearing after 48 hours of hospitalisation. Nosocomial infections can also be considered early, when they appear in the first 96 hours of hospitalisation, or late, when a process of microbial colonisation by hospital pathogens is usually involved.

2.5.1 Pneumonia

Like other infections, pneumonia can also be community or nosocomial. These types of

pneumonia differ in terms of the causative agents. Community-acquired pneumonia is generally associated with Streptococcus pneumoniae and Hemophylus influenza, mycoplasma pneumoniae, Chlamydia pneumoniae, Legionella
pneumophila, and a variety of anaerobes are also involved (ROSENTHAL and TAGER, 1975).

In nosocomial pneumonia we find the following microorganisms: gram-negative bacilli (including enteric bacilli such as Escherichia coli, Klebsiella pneumoniae, Serratia spp., Enterobacter spp, as well as Pseudomonas aeruginosa) and Staphylococcus aureus, which are the most prevalent (BENTLEY et al, 1984).

Infections are very important in the hospital environment. More than 5% of hospitalised patients develop an infection after being admitted to hospital, and pneumonia is the leading infection, affecting between 10% and 20% of cases (WENZEL, 1991). According to surveillance data from the CDC's National Nosocomial Infection Surveillance (NNIS), pneumonia is the second most common nosocomial infection overall and the most common infection in intensive care units (GEORGE, 1996). In intubated patients, the incidence of this infection is seven to twenty-one times higher than those who do not need a ventilator (MARTINO, 1998).

Several factors have been associated with the development of pneumonia or increased colonisation of the oropharynx. Host-related factors are: advanced age, malnutrition, smoking, alcoholism and intravenous drug use, as well as the severity of underlying acute or chronic pathology, previous surgery and intensive care unit admission; all of these factors significantly increase the risk of pneumonia and are not yet effective targets for prevention. The main targets for prevention are environmental sources of contamination, cross-infection by staff caring for the patient, medication and mechanical factors such as the nasogastric tube which leads to oropharyngeal colonisation and gastric reflux. The unrestricted use of antibiotics results in colonisation with nosocomial pathogens and increased antibiotic resistance. The selection of stress gastritis prophylaxis prescribed to intensive care patients has a profound effect on the risks of colonisation and infection (CRAVEN et al., 1991).

Tracheal intubation sharply reduces the natural defences of the patient's upper airways (UA) and lungs. Even with the use of modern mechanical ventilators, air quality cannot guarantee that the lower airway defence mechanisms will work effectively. Other factors such as the use of narcotics and atropine also interfere with the cough reflex and mucus viscosity, making it difficult to mobilise secretions (GROSSI and SANTOS, 1994). This nursing procedure aims to remove secretions and keep the patient's airways permeable. This procedure must be carried out following aseptic techniques, which requires exhaustive training of the nursing team. The entire nursing team is trained to perform the endotracheal suction technique following a pre-established protocol. Therefore, it can be seen in practice that many times, in the eagerness to relieve the hypersecretive patient, some steps of the endotracheal suction technique are ignored, which can add to the complications that are already inherent to the procedure, such as a drop in arterial oxygen saturation in patients who require high positive end-expiratory pressure and fraction of inspired oxygen, nosocomial pneumonia, increased intracranial pressure, atelectasis and haemodynamic instability.

There is consensus and variation on the different definitions of pneumonia. All definitions include various combinations of clinical signs and symptoms and radiological evidence, but only the Central of Disease Control (CDC) in 1988 and the European Community Nosocomial Infection Survey (EURO-NIS) include laboratory evidence, such as positive bronchial aspirate culture and positive blood culture for a particular infectious agent (CROWE and COOKE, 1998).

The criteria for diagnosing pneumonia include the presence of a new or progressive pulmonary infiltrate, fever, leucocytosis and purulent tracheobronchial secretion (MARTINO, 1998).

A time limit of forty-eight hours has been accepted as the basis for differentiating early pneumonia, which is present at the time of endotracheal intubation or develops soon after intubation, from late or true ventilator-associated pneumonia, which is neither present nor incubating at the time of intubation (MEDURI, 1993; CROWE and COOKE, 1998).

Although ventilator-associated pneumonia (VAP) can result in bacteraemia, aspiration of bacteria primarily from the oropharynx and sometimes from gastric reflux is the most important route of infection. In these patients, the flow of bacteria around the cuff of the endotracheal tube, associated with local trauma and tracheal inflammation, increases colonisation and hinders the elimination of secretions from the lower respiratory tract. Tracheal colonisation with bacteria and tracheobronchitis are common and can be precursors to VAP. Endotracheal aspiration is the main route of entry for bacteria into the lower respiratory tract (CRAVEN et al., 1991).

2.5.2 Nosocomial pneumonia

Studies show that hospitalised individuals tend not to clean their mouths satisfactorily compared to "control patients" in society (BAGRAMIAN and HELLER, 1977).

Nosocomial pneumonia is a major problem for critically ill patients in the ICU. Among the problems of pneumonia in the ICU are the diagnosis of pneumonia, the diagnosis of the etiological agent, functional alteration and initial empirical therapy. The diagnosis of pneumonia in ICU patients depends on clinical, radiological and laboratory criteria (MCKELLAR, 1985).

Costerton et al. (1995) concluded that these interactions can result from the colonisation of dental biofilm (dental plaque) by respiratory pathogens and serve as a reservoir for the colonisation of respiratory pathogens. These establish themselves in dental plaque and can be difficult to eradicate. Bacteria in dental biofilm are known to be more resistant to antibiotics than planktonic bacteria.

According to Toews (1986), there are more than 300,000 nosocomial respiratory infections a year in hospitals around the world, causing around 20,000 deaths. And these infections increase hospitalisation time by seven to nine days on average (WENZEL, 1991). The annual direct cost of diagnosing and treating nosocomial pneumonia can exceed two billion dollars (WENZEL, 1989). Hospital-acquired pneumonia is usually the result of long periods of hospitalisation, increases hospital costs and causes significant morbidity and mortality (BOYCE, 1991). Around 50 per cent of normal adults aspirate oropharyngeal contents during sleep. This aspiration occurs more frequently in individuals with altered consciousness, such as drug users, alcoholics, epileptics, or during mechanical interventions with nasogastric or endotracheal intubation. These patients tend to have a higher incidence of bacterial pneumonia than the general population. In hospitalised patients, there are four ways in which microorganisms can contaminate the lower airways: by aspiration of the contents of the oropharynx, by extension of the infection to contiguous areas, by inhalation of infected aerosols and by haematogenous dissemination to other areas of the body. Among these forms of contamination, the most common is aspiration of the contents of the oropharynx (MEGRAN and CHOW, 1986; TOEWS, 1986).

Craven et al. (1991) reported that other risk factors predispose to nosocomial pneumonia, such as chronic lung disease, congestive heart failure, diabetes mellitus, a history of smoking and immunosuppression.

In their work, Mcdonald et al. (1992) observed that pneumonia also affects a significant number of elderly people and is responsible for the majority of admissions to hospitals and wards.

According to Levison (1994), the lower airways manage to keep their sterility intact through various defence mechanisms. These include: the action of tracheobronchial secretions, the cough reflex, immune and non-immune defence factors (cell-mediated immunity, humoral immunity and polymonuclear leukocytes).

The relationship between the systemic humoral response and Prevotella species (bacteria associated with periodontal disease) and pneumonia associated with artificial ventilation of the lungs in hospitalised patients has been described. Thus, colonisation in patients by Prevotella species may be associated with infectious processes, promoting ventilation pneumonia and systemic humoral response (GROLLIER et al., 1996).

International statistics suggest that nosocomial pneumonia occurs in 5 to 10 cases per 1,000 hospital admissions and increases 6 to 20 times in patients with acute respiratory distress syndrome (ARDS), occurring in up to 70% of patients who die, although there is no direct relationship between mortality and pneumonia. Nosocomial pneumonia increases mortality (36% to 80%), especially when it is bacteraemic (DAVID, 1998).

In the ICU, the minimum criteria for a lung lesion to be considered pneumonia are: fever, purulent sputum, leucocytosis or leucopenia and new or progressive pulmonary infiltrates on chest X-ray (CONSENSO LATINO-AMERICANO DE PNEUMONIA, 1998).

The Latin American Pneumonia Consensus (1998) also states that, in addition to the minimum criteria, there are complementary methods for diagnosing nosocomial pneumonia in adult patients, such as chest X-ray, pulse oximetry or arterial blood gas, blood culture, tracheal aspirate microbiology, bacterioscopy (Gram, BAAR) and culture, pleural fluid (if present), puncture and microbiological analysis.

Although the microbiological analysis of tracheal aspirates is less sensitive, it is easier to perform and less expensive than the more refined tests that require bronchoscopy and special catheters. According to David (1998), the mortality risk attributed to nosocomial pneumonia, i.e. the percentage of deaths that would not have occurred in the absence of infection, is between 33% and 50% and varies with certain germs, being high for Pseudomonas aeruginosa, Acinetobacter calcoaceticus, methicillin-resistant S. aureus and MRSA (Methicillin-resistant Staphylococcus aureus), the latter characterised by its resistance to antibiotics. Hospital-acquired pneumonia increases the length of hospitalisation from seven (7) to nine (9) days and the cost of treatment.

Carrilho (1998), through univariate analysis, identified the following risk factors potentially involved in the genesis of hospital-acquired pneumonia: lowered level of consciousness, craniotomy surgery, previous use of antibiotics, mechanical ventilation, use of nasogastric tube, enteral diet, aspiration of gastric contents, central venous catheter and length of stay in the ICU. The final result of the analysis identified four risk factors for developing pneumonia in the ICU: tracheostomy, use of a nasogastric tube, use of an H2 blocker and lowered level of consciousness. In 32% of the patients, it was possible to identify the causative agent through protected bronchial brushings, bronchoalveolar lavage, blood culture and pleural fluid culture. The most common agents were Acinetobacter spp (33%) and S. aureus (22%). More than 56% of the patients acquired pneumonia by the fourth day of hospitalisation.

Bacteria that colonise supra- and subgingival dental plaque are cultured from saliva. These pathogenic bacteria can include those associated with periodontal disease (P. gingivalis, Fusobacterium nucleatum) or respiratory pathogens (P. aeruginosa, Klebsiella pneumoniae). Saliva is aspirated into the lower respiratory tract, where infection can occur. Cytokines from diseased periodontal tissue can enter the saliva from the gingival fluid and can also be aspirated, as well as stimulating the local inflammatory process that contributes to the onset and/or progression of infection in the lung (SCANNAPIECO et al. 1998).

According to Scannapieco et al (1992), there are phagocytic cells in the lungs that remove microorganisms and particles adhered to the respiratory mucosa. The authors reported that the possibility of oral disorders, such as periodontal disease, being a predisposing factor for nosocomial pneumonia is not ruled out. One example is hospitalised patients, especially those in the ICU, where they probably don't pay much attention to personal and oral hygiene. This neglect of oral hygiene can favour the conditions that contribute to the onset of pneumonia. According to the authors, teeth can serve as a kind of reservoir for pathogens that cause respiratory infections. In fact, this suspicion that the conditions of the oral cavity can influence the bacterial microbiota of the lower bronchi is not new.

The authors also refer to some mechanisms that can be imagined to explain how oral bacteria (P. gingivalis, A. actinomycetemcomtans) are aspirated and cause lung infection: enzymes present in saliva and associated with periodontal disease can modify the mucosal surface and promote adhesion and colonisation by respiratory pathogens; cytokines originating in periodontal tissues can alter the respiratory epithelium and promote infection by respiratory pathogens; enzymes associated with periodontal disease can destroy the salivary film over pathogenic bacteria.

Scannapieco et al. (1992) also analysed the prevalence of oral colonisation by respiratory pathogens in two groups of ICU patients. The first was characterised by patients who had been admitted to the ICU and received routine hygiene care from the professionals working there, and the second group ("control group") was represented by patients who were undergoing preventive dental care for the first time. The first examinations were carried out with special attention to dental plaque and oral mucosa over a period of two months. In the inpatient group, oral hygiene protocols were carried out and cultures taken within the first 12 hours and every three days of the patient's stay in the ICU until they were discharged or died. For patients in the so-called control group, plaque and oral mucosa cultures were only taken at the initial visit. The results of this study indicated that there was poor oral hygiene in this ICU. Approximately 65% of the plaques and oral mucosa of the selected inpatients were colonised by respiratory pathogens, in contrast to 16% of the outpatients. It was noteworthy that colonisation by respiratory pathogens was statistically associated with antibiotic therapy for ICU inpatients. The data from this study indicated that bacteria that cause nosocomial pneumonia colonise dental plaque and oral mucosa in ICU patients. In many cases, this colonisation occurs by a large number of these bacteria. Dental plaque can therefore be considered an important reservoir for these pathogens in ICU patients. Improving oral hygiene techniques in the ICU could reduce plaque colonisation and make it possible to reduce colonisation in the oropharynx.

Ziviani and Cruz (2006) compared biofilm and tracheal secretion samples from 24 patients in two groups who were being treated in an intensive care unit. After clinical examinations, oral hygiene was carried out in the first group, called the protocol group, through supervised brushing associated with the topical application of chlorhexidine once a day on all oral surfaces. This protocol was followed daily while the patient remained in the ICU. The second group, called the control group, did not receive the protocol developed for the research. Patients in the "control group" continued to receive the unit's routine hygiene care. At the end of the study, a comparative survey was carried out between the two groups to check the prevalence of dental biofilm and respiratory infections in each group. The authors concluded that simple, routine care can reduce the risk of infection in the ICU through the oral cavity. By applying the oral hygiene protocol used in this study, it was possible to reduce the rate of dental biofilm and reduce the colonisation of respiratory pathogens that cause respiratory infections, especially pneumonia.

2.6 ORAL HYGIENE FOR HOSPITALISED PATIENTS

Some patients may require suction therapy. Attention should be paid to the aggressive use of plastic suckers intended for this purpose during oral care in order to avoid oral trauma (ASHURST, 1997).

Erickson (1997) stated that toothbrushes and toothpastes combine elements that provide cleanliness and freshness to the teeth. Toothpaste formulations can contain caries control agents, preparations that prevent calculus formation, tooth sensitivity reducers and antimicrobial effects. Preference should be given to the use of fluoridated toothpastes in conjunction with toothbrushing. The use of fluoride-containing agents in varying concentrations has appropriate ratios to individual risk, so they are indicated to be part of the group of materials intended for oral care in hospitalised patients, since these mouthwashes also allow calcium fluoride to be deposited on the enamel, as well as being considered easy to apply and low cost. If adequate plaque reduction is not achieved through mechanical hygiene, the use of effective chemotherapeutic agents is indicated as long as they do not cause bacterial resistance or side effects. Chlorhexidine has antibacterial and antifungal activity. Used at a concentration of 0.12%, it is effective in inhibiting plaque formation and reducing gingivitis, has an anti-caries effect and reduces halitosis. However, it does have side effects, such as staining of the teeth and tongue, changes in the flavour of food and a reduced sense of taste. Chlorhexidine can be considered the most significant mouthwash, proving to be superior to other agents containing triclosan, phenolic derivatives or cetylpyridinium chloride in their composition. Cepacol is a cetylpyridinium chloride-based mouthwash which, despite reducing salivary bacteria, has short-lived effects. This product has been associated with the appearance of opportunistic infections such as those caused by fungi of the Candida genus. According to the author, cleaning dentures should be part of a daily care programme. Some chemical agents can facilitate the removal of plaque and stains, and the use of effervescent tablets should also be considered. Dentures should be immersed in cleaning solutions selected by the dentist in individual wide cups.

With regard to removing dentures, Erickson says that it is important to do so at night in order to preserve the integrity of the tissues and reduce bacterial proliferation, avoiding inflammation of the mucosa. However, many users remove them just to clean them. Dentures should be kept in water when not in use.

The best prevention for oral pathologies is the mechanical removal of plaque by brushing the teeth and tongue, using dental floss and other oral hygiene resources. A small toothbrush with soft bristles and rounded tips of equal height is recommended for dental hygiene (MACEDO and LACAZ NETTO, 1980).

Gastrointestinal intubation tubes are commonly used in hospitalised patients and are inserted through the mouth or nose to reach the stomach, thus influencing the patient's diet and the professional's access to the oral cavity. The nasoenteric tube is a long tube, inserted through the nose and passed through the oesophagus and stomach until it reaches the intestinal tract. Patients can stay with these materials for relatively long periods. Patients with feeding tubes used to administer diets, on the other hand, need to take essential care with oral and nasal hygiene. Maintaining the humidity of the mucous membranes is also essential, avoiding dryness and minimising discomfort (BRUNNER & SUDDARTH, 1992).

Intubated patients are forced to keep their mouths open, causing the oral mucosa to dry out (KITE and PEARSON, 1995). It is also common in ICUs to keep patients dehydrated in order to improve cardiac and respiratory function. Procedures like this can exacerbate the process of xerostomia and increase the potential for oral infections.

In an in vitro study, three commercial brands of cotton swabs and a saliva stimulator available for use in hospital environments were compared in terms of their erosive effect on tooth enamel: Dentiswab (Dentisand Pharma AB, Malmo, Sweden); Lemon- Glycerin Swabsticks (PDI, Orandeburg, NY, United States); Lemon Glycerine Swabs (Dansu A/S, Stenlose, Denmark); and the saliva stimulator Cassisal Tablets (Dentisand Pharma AB, Malmo, Sweden). An apparatus made from bovine tooth enamel was used for the research. The samples were incubated for four hours in test solutions. The results showed statistically significant enamel softening caused by two cotton swabs, "Lemon-Glycerin Swabsticks" and "Lemon Glycerine Swabs". Incubation in solutions made with "Dentiswab" and "Cassisal Tablets" caused minimal changes to the enamel samples selected for the study and, for this reason, these were the products indicated for cleaning the oral cavity (MEURMAN et al., 1996).

Any signs of oral infections detected by nurses should be referred for appropriate treatment. Therefore, it is more appropriate for signs and symptoms of oral pathologies to be identified in advance by dental professionals at the time of the patient's hospitalisation (GOLDIE et al., 1996).

Potter and Perry (1999) highlight the frequent referral of hospitalised patients for dental examinations and treatment. It should be emphasised that regular examinations are also necessary to prevent oral cancer (ERICKSON, 1997).

The formation of plaque on dentures serves as a substrate for Candida albicans. Hospitalised patients should be given further instructions on mucosal inflammation and prosthesis hygiene. Several studies have shown that hospitalised patients have difficulty retaining dentures due to decreased salivation (TURANO and TURANO, 1998). The interruption in the use of prosthetic rehabilitations generates changes in the mucosa, induces resorption of the alveolar bone and reduces the vertical dimension of occlusion (VOD). Patients who don't wear prostheses have more pronounced facial furrows and an apparently "withered" face, the chin is positioned forwards and closer to the apex of the nose, the position of the lips changes and the facial appearance becomes aged. The absence of prostheses, as well as affecting function and aesthetics, alters phonetics and has psychological implications, discouraging social interaction. The use of complete dentures is known to help maintain the health of adjacent supporting structures and restore masticatory capacity, depending on the motivation for use and hygiene. In short, the use of prostheses whenever possible in the hospital environment improves the general health condition of patients.

Although aware of the need for oral intubation to maintain breathing and life in some ICU patients, Barnason et al (1998) reported that this procedure can often cause significant changes in their recovery. In the case of severe illnesses, bacteria that are naturally present in the oral cavity, which are predominantly gram-positive, can become gram-negative, thus increasing their potential for infection.

Manual toothbrushes should be selected according to the patient's needs, and can be used with appropriate and individualised frequencies. Oral care with conventional toothbrushes may not be effective for patients with lower motor and cognitive skills, and the use of toothbrushes with modified handles that facilitate grip is recommended, as well as electric rotary/oscillatory brushes that rescue remaining skills. However, when adequate hygiene is not possible using only toothbrushes with bristles, hospitalised patients can also use foam brushes combined with chlorhexidine solutions to clean mucous membranes. In Brazil, these brushes are not widespread. We have, however, found wooden sticks wrapped in gauze as substitutes. It is believed that oral hygiene protocols carried out by nursing teams can be easily modified in relation to what has been used to apply therapeutic agents. It should be emphasised that the conventional method is still considered the most effective for cleaning the oral cavity, especially when combined with the use of mouthwashes containing fluoride agents. Moisturising the lips with water-soluble creams is also recommended (POTTER and PERRY, 1999).

The intubated patient may need a Guedel cannula, a semi-circular instrument, usually made of plastic and disposable, which, when properly placed, displaces the tongue from the posterior pharyngeal wall, keeping the airway open. Before inserting the cannula, secretions and blood clots in the mouth and pharynx must be removed by suction, as well as movable dentures. If the cannula is placed incorrectly, it can dislodge the tongue into the pharynx and obstruct the airway. To avoid injury to the patient, the resuscitator must ensure that the lips and tongue do not come between the cannula and the teeth (ALEXANDRE & BRITO, 2000). The authors also suggested that when removing debris from the mouth in dependent patients, a 1% bicarbonate solution should be used with wooden spatulas wrapped in gauze to aid cleaning.

Another factor to consider in relation to the oral health of intubated patients is the impact of the use of drugs or the procedures required to treat their medical condition that cause damage to the oral cavity, such as xerostomia (MCNEILL, 2000).

In hospitals, the destabilisation of a patient's organ system caused by the presence of a new pathology, the exacerbation of a chronic pathology or complications during surgical procedures can result in the need to be admitted to intensive care units (ICUs). ICUs have the function of grouping critically ill patients together for better observation, reducing mortality through continuous and comprehensive individual care according to specific needs. In unconscious patients, oral hygiene care cannot be neglected and needs to be carried out more frequently, as these patients do not salivate when faced with reactions involving sight, smell and food intake. Dry crusts containing mucus, microorganisms and desquamated cells are also frequently seen on the lips and teeth of these patients, which can be removed using a mixture of sodium bicarbonate and saline solution. Tooth brushing is preferred, but precautions are needed to avoid aspiration of fluids. Hospitalised patients suffering from dental problems can have their discomfort alleviated with guidance from nurses and carers, through hygiene and prevention in the institution. During their hospitalisation they can develop, among other illnesses, stomatitis, especially those undergoing chemotherapy or radiotherapy or intubated with a nasogastric tube (SOUZA et al., 2001).

Epstein et al. (2001) stated that benzydamine hydrochloride, known as Tantum, is effective when used during the oral hygiene of ICU patients, as it has anti-inflammatory, analgesic and antibacterial properties. When applied prophylactically, this product shows better results than when used therapeutically, when mucositis is present. However, in some cases studied, Tantum also appears as an aggressive agent, causing a sensation of numbness or burning in the oral soft tissues.

Poor or unsatisfactory oral hygiene has been the cause of tooth loss (BROOK et al., 2002) and dentistry has made great strides in the scientific field of oral hygiene (GADBURY-AMYOT et al, 2002), preventing most oral pathologies from occurring and minimising the effects of oral diseases that have already set in.

In a cross-sectional study at the national hospital in Chubu, Japan, a strong association was observed between certain factors, such as the ability to self-feed, the inability to rinse mouth, not eating at the table, severe dementia, and the frequency of tooth brushing. Patients who had lost the ability to eat were unable to maintain their own oral hygiene. In addition to the routine care of feeding devices, which has previously been recognised as necessary, attention should be paid to oral hygiene procedures in order to prevent the occurrence of dental diseases and fatal pneumonia in patients (ARAI et al, 2003).

Most causes of bad breath come from bacterial proteolytic activity in the mouth. The bacteria predominantly present on the tongue of individuals with halitosis are identified as those that contribute most to the presence of the odour (KAZOR et al., 2003). Thus, cleaning the tongue is of paramount importance for oral hygiene and quality of life. This care, especially in bedridden patients, is necessary due to the large bacterial presence in this region, which can present a risk of pulmonary contamination, which is of real importance. Tongue cleaners are, in this case, efficient means of health care and should be widely used (LEITE, 2005).

Patients with tooth loss or total edentulism should receive proper hygiene and care for their dentures. As for its maintenance in the hospital environment, nurses should encourage patients to sanitise it frequently. Suitable brushes and toothpaste are recommended for hygiene of the gums, palate and tongue. Brushes made for cleaning complete dentures (PTMS) and brushes for removable partial dentures (PPR) help to clean these appliances more effectively, but are still little known (LAURIA et al, 2003).

After removing the intubation, oral hygiene should be carried out in bed with the aid of an emesis bucket, the act of expelling secretions from the oral cavity. This hygiene practice helps to contain the formation of bacterial plaque during the proper replacement of removable dentures. In this sense, once the patient has favourable conditions, they will be able to chew better and ingest essential nutrients. Preventive care can be carried out after intubation has been removed, as well as by instructing the nursing team (BRUNETTI & MONTENEGRO, 2003).

Still on the subject of the need for treatment and hygiene care in hospitalised patients, Peltola et al. (2004), in a cross-sectional study, through clinical oral examinations of elderly patients, with an average age of 83.3 years, hospitalised for long periods, observed that 42% of these were edentulous; 41% had their prostheses removed by the professional team during hospitalisation. As for the hygiene of the prostheses worn by the patients, 19% were classified as adequate, 44% were classified as having moderate hygiene quality and 37% were included in the poor hygiene group. Within the group of denture wearers, stomatitis was found in 25% of the patients examined and angular cheilitis in 28% of them. Oral hygiene was therefore considered unsatisfactory. In the group of denture wearers, 37 per cent needed restorations, 51 per cent required periodontal therapy and 42 per cent needed tooth extractions. It was concluded that greater attention should be paid to oral health care in elderly patients hospitalised for longer periods, establishing daily professional aids during oral hygiene procedures.

In ICUs, dentists can accompany nursing staff, assist the family, ensure careful intubation in the presence of natural teeth and clean the oral cavity using solutions such as chlorhexidine (ABIDIA, 2004).

Flossing is necessary for the effective removal of plaque between the teeth and should be used after brushing. It is up to the nurse to encourage this habit and demonstrate the appropriate methods for holding the floss and cleaning these areas. Cylindrical or conical interdental brushes for cleaning spaces between teeth are effective during oral hygiene. When the patient has a larger area to be cleaned, or has fixed dentures, the so-called floss threaders or adapted floss make it easier to floss the areas near the gums. Wooden toothpicks, on the other hand, can cause damage to the gums. Some modified plastic toothpicks have been introduced onto the market, but no studies have been found to prove that they are effective or less harmful than conventional wooden toothpicks (REZENDE, 2005).

The assessment of hospitalised patients should cover the history and physical assessment of the oral cavity during anamnesis, observing all the structures in the mouth, detecting the presence of any alterations to normality, such as infections, chemical or mechanical trauma and pain. The professional should also assess the colour of the mucous membranes, the shape, volume and contour of the structures oral, as well as the conditions of hygiene and dental treatment present. It is essential that the patient keeps their mouth meticulously clean and that the nursing staff instructs them on the importance and techniques of preventive oral care (SAFDAR et al., 2005).

Oral hygiene is considered a basic procedure for teams of professionals working in intensive care units. Care should be intensified for those patients who require mechanical ventilation, as the endotracheal intubation to which they are subjected facilitates bacterial adherence to the mucosa, in addition to the influence of drugs that cause xerostomia, which are often administered to these types of patients, causing damage to the oral cavity (DEPUYDT et al., 2006). The primary aim of oral care is to minimise the formation of dental plaque and the accumulation of debris in the oropharynx, which creates an ideal environment for pathogenic microorganisms that cause diseases such as stomatitis and gingivitis. In this context, oral care can effectively maintain oral health and reduce the incidence of pneumonia in patients requiring mechanical ventilation (KOEMAN et al., 2001)

For Abidia (2007), an important point to consider is the impact of unfavourable nutritional status on the oral cavity. Orally intubated patients have to be fed artificially, via the enteral or parenteral route, since they are unable to swallow by mouth. Among other issues related to oral care in ICUs, the author discussed the importance of nutrition for ICU patients and pointed to reduced recovery power and decreased immunity to infections among the main consequences of inadequate nutrition.

Despite the apparent advantages gained from carrying out proper oral care in ICU patients, it can be seen that this subject still does not receive enough attention. Little information is found in the literature on current practices, training, perceptions and attitudes of ICU professionals towards oral care for their patients. According to the authors, there is a need to evaluate different types of oral hygiene protocols for intubated patients. Conclusion reached after comparing different tracheal intubation techniques with regard to the promotion of oral hygiene techniques in these patients. Intubation and oral hygiene techniques should be selected according to the individual characteristics of each patient who needs them (RELLO et al, 2007).

Hur et al. (2007) explored the effect of an essential oil solution of "tea tree" in combating bad odour and volatile sulphur components, which are the main components responsible for the occurrence of bad breath in the oral cavity of ICU patients in South Korea. Also called "malaleuca", this product has been known for hundreds of years by Australian tribes of Bundialung Aborigines, and its main characteristics are that it acts as an antiseptic in two ways: through a direct action on microorganisms, and secondly through a process of activating white blood cells in the body's defence process. This product is considered to have immunostimulant properties, which makes it a formidable alternative for patients with low resistance and/or diseases that weaken their immunology and allow untimely illnesses to appear, even in cases where the most commonly used antibiotics fail. In this study, two qualified nurses performed three-minute oral hygiene procedures on 32 ICU patients. Teeth, tongue and oral cavity were cleaned with gauze soaked in "tea tree" solution on the first day of the study and with Tantum on the second day. Visual analogue scales, to measure bad odour, and a "Halimeter", a device used in the doctor's office capable of diagnosing and quantifying bad breath, were used in the study. The differences between the two products were quite significant. The findings suggest that the tea tree solution is an efficient method for reducing bad odour and volatile sulphur components in ICU patients.

The importance of oral hygiene for the well-being, prevention of systemic diseases and better recovery of ICU patients is not well publicised in Brazil. MORAIS et al (2007), who started providing dental care in the ICU of the Santa Casa de Misericórdia de Barretos, São Paulo, five years ago, when they noticed the lack of this service, and who today form the coordination team of the hospital's dental department, say that many studies report that few Brazilian hospitals have a dental hygienist integrated into the unit's multidisciplinary team, or nurses who are trained and orientated on appropriate oral hygiene methods for patients in these conditions. For the authors, one of the main reasons for this negligence is that, even with the evolution of knowledge, medicine still gives little importance to oral problems and has not incorporated the benefits that caring for the stomatognathic system brings to the patient. "For over 150 years, hand hygiene has been the most important measure for controlling hospital-acquired infections. But so far, a source of infection as important as the mouth, considered a favourable environment for microbial growth, has been overlooked," say the authors. On the other hand, it must also be considered that many dental professionals are not prepared to work in the ICU, as they are unaware of the medical aspects related to their work. "Doctors and dental surgeons need to integrate their knowledge in order to fully manage patients, especially critically ill patients, and provide them with quality of life," they conclude. Patients in the ICU require special and complex care from the professionals around them. As well as having sufficient technical and scientific knowledge to treat oral problems that could complicate the case in a way that suits the possibilities and limitations of these patients, the DS must have good knowledge of Basic Life Support (BLS), which includes basic first aid procedures in cardiac emergencies. The authors also state that at Santa Casa de Barretos, in the state of São Paulo, training courses in oral hygiene are held periodically for the ICU team, given by a dental surgeon. In addition, the entire multidisciplinary team of the unit meets weekly to discuss the health condition of each patient and together determine the treatment plan. Dentistry is always included in the strategies drawn up within the hospital to control hospital-acquired infections.

Regarding oral hygiene procedures, the authors state that, in addition to removing bacterial plaque, dental care should also aim to relieve pain and discomfort in the mouth, prevent accidents related to the oral cavity and provide health education for patients and the entire multi-professional ICU team.

However, mechanical procedures can't always be carried out efficiently, as oral hygiene procedures are beneficial not only to inpatients, but also to the hospital itself, which has its costs reduced. Difficulties in improving the clinical condition and the consequent worsening of the prognosis prolong the patient's stay in the ICU and reduce the possibility of vacancies, increasing hospital costs. It should also be emphasised that dental care in the ICU involves irrelevant expenses, as these are simple and inexpensive procedures that provide great benefits. Currently, many hospitals use various resources to combat the large volume of bacteria in the oropharynx, one of the main causes of hospital respiratory infections, such as the administration and topical application of antibiotics, respiratory physiotherapy, oxygen therapy and other preventative measures. However, these methods are not only more expensive than practising oral hygiene, they are also more harmful to the patient, as they increase the risk of microorganism resistance in the case of medication. Research indicates that controlling the dental biofilm of critically ill patients can be done at least three times a day. According to the conclusion of their study, the work can be done either by a dental surgeon, by a THD under the supervision of a CD, or by the nursing assistant themselves, as long as they are trained and supervised by the CD.

2.7 KNOWLEDGE AND ACTIONS OF THE NURSING TEAM ON ORAL HEALTH

Oral hygiene techniques administered by nurses are found in select scientific articles in the fields of medicine and dentistry. According to a study carried out in 1985, the importance of oral hygiene for nursing staff is a consequence of physiological, pathophysiological, psychosocial, epidemiological and economic perspectives. According to the literature review analysed (ROTH and CREASON, 1986), there is no standard for the oral care techniques performed by nurses. While some authors claim that just using swabs soaked in antiseptic solutions is enough to maintain the health of patients' oral cavities, others claim that without brushing teeth and tongue it would be impossible to avoid the onset and worsening of certain pathologies related to other vital organs of the body. The presence of an oral health professional in clinics and hospitals would be of the utmost importance, since it would be up to them to guide and monitor whether these procedures are being carried out successfully.

Liwu (1990) conducted a prospective study in an intensive care unit. The aim was to analyse the health and incidence of infection in the oral mucous membranes of 40 totally dependent inpatients who required mechanical ventilation. In 50% of these patients, oral care consisted of applying swabs soaked in mouthwash containing 0.5% cetylpyridinium chloride and 17% ethanes (Ultrafresh), a routine procedure in ICUs. In the other group of patients, the use of saline solution replaced the mouthwash in the first group. Patients suffering from periodontal disease were excluded from the study and edentulous patients made up 65% of the sample. The condition of oral mucosa tissues and dental elements was recorded before and after intubation, two weeks later, according to pre-selected criteria. There were no significant differences between the efficacy of the two solutions used in the study. The soft tissues analysed continued to look healthy. The appearance of ulcerations analysed in the patients' tissues and lips was related to the pressure exerted by the positioning of the endotracheal tubes. It is worth noting that these procedures were considered ineffective for removing debris that was located between dental elements and in the tongue region.

Logan et al. (1991), in their study with nurses, hospital directors and home care nurses, found several misconceptions about dental care practices in hospitalised patients. The lack of knowledge about dental pathologies was found to be wide-ranging, covering numerous aspects such as examining the oral cavity, characteristics of cancer lesions, oral hygiene care, cleaning dentures, xerostomia and other side effects of medication. Patients' mobility difficulties and other physical limitations are seen as the biggest obstacles or impossibilities to dental care. It was estimated that 48 per cent of the professionals who took part in the survey had not had access to this knowledge and 30 per cent of the sample demonstrated that this was not a priority issue in their work. The authors suggest that in training programmes for nursing staff, teachings related to dental care should be addressed to these professionals, instructing them about possible dental pathologies present that are commonly related to systemic diseases.

The United Kingdom Central Council's (UKCC) Code of Conduct for Nurses (1992) requires nurses to act at all times with the aim of promoting patient safety and well-being, as well as ensuring that no act or omission within nurses' sphere of responsibility is carried out. The code also establishes that nursing professionals must provide individualised care and actions according to the needs of each patient they assist.

Usually, nursing teams treating critically ill patients have the responsibility of planning and applying some types of basic oral care. However, oral hygiene practices carried out by nurses have been defined as inconsistent and often variable, with no standardised protocols. Treating the oropharynx and maintaining favourable hygiene are difficult procedures to carry out in very sick patients, especially those on mechanical ventilation due to the difficult access to the oral cavity. Intubated patients are at greater risk of being colonised by microorganisms, as the oral cavity is in contact with other instruments such as tapes, mouthpieces, tubes, among others (TREOLAR and STECHMILLER, 1995). The function of the oral endotracheal tube is to provide ventilation and protection for the passage of air. The position of the tube and other support materials can obstruct visualisation of the oral cavity and limit access, negatively influencing the hygiene process. As a result, nursing professionals are reluctant to manipulate the apparatus necessary for patients to breathe in order to carry out hygiene procedures. In turn, fixation tapes present too close to the oral cavity quickly become heavily contaminated with pathogens when saliva molecules are manipulated in an attempt to carry out hygiene techniques (HAYES and JONES, 1995).

Moore (1995) concluded that the graduate schools and institutions in which these nursing professionals work should review the basic oral hygiene criteria administered by these teams and that new standards for these techniques need to be carefully planned, applied and evaluated. The author pointed out that in the 29 years prior to his research, there had been few or almost no changes in oral hygiene practices carried out in hospital environments.

Questionnaires on knowledge and actions relating to oral care for critically ill patients were used to interview nursing professionals working in this area. It was concluded that the use of a standard protocol to guide these nurses during oral care procedures would significantly improve the quality of the procedures and make it easier to record what was being done. The questionnaires contained 29 objective questions to facilitate data tabulation. 70 professionals were invited to take part, but only 34 returned the completed interviews. Among other results, it was confirmed that: nursing teams were interested in receiving more and up-to-date information on oral hygiene; the sample size was considered small; the professionals assessed did not have sufficient knowledge of oral hygiene techniques to provide adequate oral care for their patients (WASH et al, 2004).

Patients in ICUs need very specific care, which requires the presence of highly qualified professionals. It is often noted that the oral care provided by these professionals to their patients is considered a low priority by ICU teams as well as in nursing training programmes. However, the importance and benefits of these procedures have been emphasised and presented worldwide. Observing and recording individual oral care needs should be considered mandatory procedures upon admission to hospital (LONGHURST, 1998).

With regard to the technical training of carers, it is the dentist's job to present basic preventive treatment techniques for oral diseases to nursing professionals who are in direct contact with patients. With regard to nursing care for elderly patients, nursing professionals should have positive attitudes, enabling their patients' independence and self-esteem, thus promoting more effective care (POTTER and PERRY, 1999).

In a study, Fitch et al. (1999) tested the use of an oral care protocol in ICUs. The procedures promoted by this protocol were carried out by nurses and had very different characteristics to what had been done routinely up to that point. Firstly, paediatric brushes were used, which had the advantage of being small enough to remove plaque without influencing the position of the ventilation tube. Their soft bristles reduced the risk of trauma and bleeding. The products of choice selected were antibacterial and did not contain alcohol in order to sanitise without drying out the membranes of the oral mucosa. Although the author used the commercial brand "Biotene", other antimicrobials can be suggested, such as "Perioaid" (VAN STRYDONCK et al., 2005) or "Crest Pro-Health Mouthrinse" (WHITE, 2005). In the same study, Oral Balance oral moisturisers were applied to the patients' mucous membranes, and petroleum jelly, a product similar to Vaseline, was applied to the lips to reduce dryness. The nurses were able to carry out all the procedures guided by the protocol in less than five minutes and agreed that this new oral care routine would be more effective in treating their patients. The experimental protocol was effective in reducing inflammation, while the care previously carried out did not prove effective for these changes. It was concluded that protocols applied to nursing teams are capable of improving the health of ICU patients. Positive correlations were also recorded for saliva appearance, bleeding and halitosis. This study also affirmed that members of the nursing team can effectively perform oral hygiene care on ICU patients, provided they have access to appropriate training with a specialised dental professional.

Thirty-four members of nursing teams working in hospitals were interviewed about the oral care provided to elderly inpatients (ADAMS, 1996). Questionnaires containing 29 questions aimed at the target audience were used and a due date was set. Among the conclusions reached, the following stand out: the use of a standardised protocol for oral hygiene procedures would increase the quality of hygiene carried out up to that point; the professionals interviewed were interested in acquiring more knowledge about oral health and care for their patients; and there was a lack of adequate knowledge about patients' oral health on the part of the nursing teams interviewed in this study.

Blank et al. (1996) found that 83% of the nursing staff had not received basic training in oral health. The researchers emphasise the need to improve the quality of oral care for geriatric patients and conclude that appropriate training and the presence of a dentist in the hospital environment contribute to improved knowledge and better nursing performance in relation to patients' oral health.

Mcneill (2000) concluded that health professionals caring for intubated patients need to know perfectly how to carry out oral hygiene procedures in order to prevent the development or worsening of certain diseases and promote the best possible well-being of their patients. Therefore, during the preparation of these professionals, greater importance should be given to the care and recognition of oral pathologies in intubated patients, as this is a complex and difficult procedure to carry out. The development of oral hygiene protocols for these types of patients should also be better developed and standardised in schools preparing nursing teams.

Wall et al. (2001) state that advances in the organisation and management of patients in ICUs have ensured reductions in the morbidity and mortality of severely ill patients. Two of the biggest advances include the participation of multidisciplinary teams and the development of clinical protocols. The use of protocols by these teams does not guarantee an immediate improvement in the quality of care provided, but they do offer useful tools capable of achieving these goals, if they are applied correctly by professionals from different areas, specialities and sub-specialities with a single objective: the patient's well-being.

In 2003, Grap et al. interviewed 170 members of staff and patients who responded to a survey aimed at describing the frequency of use of oral care by nursing staff in severely debilitated patients admitted to intensive care units and rooms in hospitals in the United States. The majority of respondents, 75 per cent, reported that actual care was carried out two or three times a day in non-intubated patients, and 72 per cent of respondents said that in intubated patients, care of the oral cavity was carried out five or more times a day, but this is not documented in medical records. It was also recorded that the use of toothpaste and toothbrushes is significantly higher in non-intubated patients and the use of gauze wrapped around a wooden stick is more evident in patients using mechanical ventilation. Oral care in the ICU was prioritised at 53.9 on a scale of 0 to 100, according to the nursing teams interviewed. According to the results of this study, although there is scientific evidence that wooden sticks wrapped in gauze are inefficient at removing plaque, these utensils are still favoured for oral care in the ICU. Despite the existence of important utensils that can be used for oral care in ICUs, they are rarely used. Among the reasons given for not using such tools, the lack of time or lack of knowledge on the part of the professional responsible and the lack of assistance from specialised oral health professionals within the ICU were the most frequently reported. Interactions with dental hygienists could improve the knowledge and skills of the nursing staff in relation to oral care. Historically, there has been no interest in bringing in dental professionals to treat ICU patients or to advise nursing staff on oral care practices or the prevention of oral pathologies (ABIDIA, 2004).

Jones et al. (2004) researched the priority given to oral care and the knowledge and attitudes of the professionals responsible for these procedures in ICUs. 160 questionnaires were distributed to 160 nurses working in adult ICUs. In summary, oral care was prioritised in the same way as other routine procedures. 13.5 per cent of respondents considered oral care to be a low priority. 98% of the professionals performed oral hygiene on their patients and only 26% followed a protocol for recording these treatments. Toothbrushes are used at least once a day by 85.5% of the nurses and products containing chlorhexidine are routinely used by 50.5% of the survey's target audience. 23.5% of the nurses had not had any specific training in oral care and 58% claimed to be interested in better professional preparation for this purpose. It was concluded that most of the oral care methods surveyed were adequate. A small minority of the population interviewed considered oral procedures to be of low priority and did not respect existing ICU protocols. Encouraging the performance of these procedures in ICUs is a priority, as is more specific training for professionals.

Binkley et al. (2004), after interviewing 566 professionals, 97% of whom were nurses, in 102 ICUs in the United States, found that 92% of those interviewed considered oral care to be a high priority procedure in ICUs. The first methods of choice for oral care, according to the results of this survey, are swabs, mouth moisturisers and mouthwash. Brushes and toothpaste are used by approximately 80 per cent of the professionals surveyed. The vast majority of nurses showed an interest in improving their scientific knowledge on the subject. It was concluded that oral care in ICUs does not follow a standardised protocol. The current oral hygiene procedures used by the hospitals in question are inefficient in removing plaque and respiratory pathogens from the oropharynx in intubated patients. More efficient oral hygiene procedures, which include tooth brushing and the use of antimicrobial solutions, have been shown to improve the patient's oral health and can significantly reduce respiratory infections in intubated patients. More studies on this subject are needed in order to change the current oral care interventions in ICUs and, consequently, improve the quality of care in these units, reducing the incidence of ventilator-associated pneumonia.

Reviewing mentions of assessment, treatment of dental diseases and oral hygiene care found in nursing literature, few references were available. The books and articles researched are generally of foreign origin. In the countries of origin, the health professional responsible for this care is the doctor, with subsequent training in stomatology (REZENDE, 2005).

Hanneman et al. (2005) collected data on procedures for elevating the patient's head position and oral care carried out by nursing staff with the aim of reducing the risk of aspiration pneumonia in ICUs. A total of 181 questionnaires were completed and 436 beds were observed. The results showed differences in the products used for oral hygiene and the frequency of these procedures in intubated patients, four times a day, and in those who did not need mechanical ventilation, three times a day. The use of mouthwash, toothbrushes and dentifrices was higher in non-intubated patients. Swabs moistened with chlorhexidine and sodium chloride solutions were the instruments of choice most of the time in intubated patients. However, it was noted that the frequency of procedures reported by the professionals was often higher than those recorded in the patients' medical records, jeopardising the reliability of their responses. As for the elevation of the patients' head position, those who needed mechanical ventilation had their head elevated by 23° and for non-intubated patients the chosen elevation height was 30°.

Cutler and Davis (2005) observed the oral treatment that intubated patients received from the nursing staff in ICUs. The researchers spent a total of 172 hours in contact with staff and patients in

08 ICUs. In all, 253 patients were observed. The study was divided into three distinct phases. During the first phase, the routine followed by the nursing team with regard to oral hygiene was observed. It was noted that there was no protocol on frequency or instruments to be used that were followed by the professionals. The second phase of the research was marked by a training session given to the ICU nursing staff. A protocol developed by the researchers was presented to be tested during patients' oral hygiene, hygiene kits were assembled to be used during oral care, and 30 days was the time needed to prepare the team. Subsequently, procedures following the new suggested protocol were carried out by the professionals who had received the instructions. In the first phase, it was noted that oral hygiene was carried out using swabs moistened with sodium bicarbonate and a 1.5% hydrogen peroxide solution. None of the patients observed had their teeth brushed. Significant improvements were observed in all aspects during the post-training observation phase in which brushing techniques, suction of secretions and moisturisation of oral tissues were used every two hours. They concluded that applying an oral hygiene protocol improves the quality of procedures performed on intubated patients. Frequent training ensures that the nursing team is prepared to carry out procedures more safely and efficiently, thus improving the well-being and health of patients.

After reviewing the literature, Berry and Davidson (2006) concluded that there is no definitive evidence on the best hygiene method, including mouthwash. Some obstacles that prevented success during this procedure in ICU patients were identified in this research, such as equipment and mechanical barriers, perceptions of the importance of oral care on the part of the nursing staff, patient dependence and discomfort, and communication difficulties with the patient. The authors concluded that the use of a specific protocol for oral care implemented within these units would be an excellent tool for improving the quality of these procedures. They suggested that further studies be carried out on the subject with the aim of guiding and informing nursing staff about dental activities in hospitals, especially in ICUs, given the inability of these professionals to master appropriate techniques.

Researchers from the University of Louisville, USA, designed a questionnaire containing twenty-seven questions with the aim of developing a survey to verify different forms and frequency of oral care practices carried out in European ICUs as well as the perceptions and knowledge about oral hygiene of their professionals. Due to the lack of similar studies developed and tested previously, the interview was based on a review of the literature on the following questions: a) What types and frequency of oral care are provided to patients in ICUs? b) What are the attitudes and perceptions of professionals working in ICUs about oral hygiene? c) What type of training on oral care is given to these people? After being tested in the country of origin, fifty-nine questionnaires were distributed among members of the European Society of Intensive Care Medicine representing ICUs in eight countries: Spain (n=33), Greece (n=12), France (n=5), Belgium (n=3), Italy (n=3), Germany (n=1), Andorra (n=1) and Turkey (n=1). As a result, the researchers found that 77 per cent of respondents said they had received adequate training in ICU oral care. The most common oral care practice demonstrated by the study population was the use of chlorhexidine mouthwashes at least once a day. The majority of interviewees believe that nurses should be responsible for oral cavity hygiene in intubated patients, while the minority agreed that a dentist should carry out this procedure. As for the instruments used for oral care, 81 per cent reported that they had adequate equipment. However, 63 per cent said that better equipment was needed for such procedures to be carried out in ICUs. Only a third of the participants said that the toothbrushes provided by the hospital were adequate, but 37 per cent said that toothbrushes were not available, somewhat contradicting the previous statement. 27 per cent preferred electric toothbrushes to manual ones. It was concluded that oral care is of great importance in European ICUs and is generally carried out by nurses. These procedures are considered difficult to carry out. More attention should be paid to the use of toothbrushes, which are considered to be highly effective in hygiene, but are rarely found in the ICUs that took part in the study (RELLO et al., 2007).

CHAPTER 3

PROPOSAL

The aim of this study was to assess the perceptions and actions of the nursing team regarding the oral health care provided to patients admitted to Intensive Care Units during the daily oral hygiene process to which they have been subjected.

CHAPTER 4

MATERIALS AND METHODS

4.1 MATERIALS

- Questionnaire prepared in the Microsoft Office Word 2007 programme, printed on two sheets of A4 paper;
- One thousand two hundred and six (1,206) sheets of A4 paper, weight 75mg/m2, with photocopies of the questionnaire stapled to them, totalling four hundred and two (402) questionnaires;
- Ten (10) BIC ballpoint pens for the answers;
- Acrylic clipboard for conducting the interviews;
- Thirteen (13) letters of introduction signed by the supervisor of the research project, on the letterhead of the Federal University of Pará;
- Thirteen (13) white, letter-size envelopes for storing, transporting and delivering the cover letters;
- Microsoft Excel 2007 software for data tabulation and statistical analysis;
- SPSS 13.0 for Windows Vista software for data tabulation and statistical analysis;

4.2 METHODS

In order to obtain a profile of the perception and performance of oral care by nursing staff, a survey was carried out using a statistical approach to analysing data, involving as a reference population nursing professionals who worked in intensive care units of public and private hospitals located in the city of Belém, between June and November 2007. It should be made clear that the institutions considered were those with intensive care units for adult patients and which had at least eight beds available for use.

After investigating the number of public and private institutions that met the established criteria, 13 hospitals were found to meet the required profile. Of the thirteen existing institutions, twelve were visited and agreed to take part in the research. One institution, through a statement from its board of directors, refused to take part in the study and did not give a reason for its lack of interest. Aware of the existence of hospitals that treated both private and public patients, it was decided not to divide them into different groups, since comparing public and private hospitals was not the aim of the study and dividing them into groups would compromise the accuracy and coherence of the results.

The study population was made up of professionals who were part of the nursing teams working in the intensive care units of the selected institutions, divided into three training categories: nurses, nursing technicians and nursing assistants (BRASIL, 1987).

After being submitted to and approved by the human research ethics committee of the health sciences centre of the Federal University of Pará, the research was then carried out using a questionnaire containing a personal interview conducted by a single interviewer, a dental surgeon (SECCO & PEREIRA, 2004).

A total of 402 nursing professionals of both sexes, with no age limits, who worked in 23 intensive care units belonging to 12 public and private health institutions in Belém, the capital of the state of Pará, were interviewed.

Firstly, for thirty days, the ICU of one of the participating hospitals was visited daily in random shifts by the interviewer, duly introduced to the head nurse, wearing a lab coat and identification badge, with the aim of familiarising himself with the routine of the procedures carried out and making sure that the proposed study was valid. Within this first phase, 10 professionals were invited to answer the questionnaires, characterising the pilot test of this research. These interviewees were informed of the need to participate again in the future. The availability of the professionals, the time needed to complete the questionnaire, frequent questions and statistical tests to analyse the data obtained were all successfully observed.

The questionnaire was formulated with 18 multiple choice questions. This number was determined in an attempt to mention the most significant issues, thus avoiding delays, since the professionals would be at work and would not have much time to answer the document in question. The average time of the interviews was timed in advance and it was recorded that approximately four minutes and thirty seconds would be needed for each chosen member to take part.

The first part of the questionnaire, represented by questions 01 to 07, aimed to assess the profile of the nursing staff interviewed in terms of professional category, age group, gender, income, type of institution in which they work and their training.

The following questions referred to participation in a multidisciplinary team, contact or not with a dental surgeon and the nursing team's level of knowledge regarding dentistry and its relationship with the individual's general health.

Question 12 was used to assess the knowledge and care that is actually given to patients during their stay in hospital. Finally, question 18 assessed the nursing staff's level of interest in receiving guidance on oral health and applying it clinically.

Once they had the research project, the approximate number of interviewees and participating institutions and the questionnaire duly formatted, a team of professionals from the Centre for Exact and Natural Sciences, Department of Statistics, at the Federal University of Pará, under the coordination of Prof. Dr. Maria Regina Madruga Tavares, was consulted and invited to take part in the analysis with the aim of directing the best statistical tests that would meet the needs of the research, thus avoiding any possible inaccuracies during the subsequent tabulation of data and analysis of the results obtained.

To administer the questionnaire, the interviewer visited the hospitals carrying a letter drawn up by the research project's supervisor, Prof Dr Adriano Maia Corrêa, offering to explain the objectives of the study. After receiving a positive opinion from the hospital board authorising the interviews, the questionnaires were handed out individually to the nursing staff. The professional was expected to answer the questions and any doubts were solved by the interviewer, ensuring that the interviewees gave conscious and confident answers. It is important to mention that visits to the hospitals took place during all shifts (morning, afternoon and evening), following work schedules established by each hospital. It was necessary to return to the institutions when it was noticed that not all the professionals working at the time were present, in order to approach all the nursing teams. Professionals who were on holiday or on professional leave were not included in our reports as part of the study's target audience. The selected interviewees were informed of the non-obligatory nature of their participation by means of a free and informed consent form, as well as the guarantee of absolute confidentiality in relation to their identity and the name of the workplace in which they worked.

4.3 STATISTICAL TESTS

With regard to the statistical tests selected for this study, we used the proportion test. The aim of this test is to compare the proportion of individuals with a given characteristic, obtained from the sample, with a proportion p. The hypothesis we tested in this work is whether the proportion of individuals with a given characteristic is equal to 0.5. This hypothesis is called the null hypothesis (Ho). There is also another hypothesis in question, which contradicts the null hypothesis, called the alternative hypothesis (H1). If the null hypothesis is rejected, then we accept the alternative hypothesis as true. The method used to analyse this test is the p-value.

Summary of the test used:

1) The hypotheses are defined.

The null hypothesis will always be that the proportion p of individuals with a given characteristic is equal to 0.5.

The alternative hypothesis could be:

a) The proportion p is different from 0.5;
b) The p-ratio is greater than 0.5;
c) The proportion p is less than 0.5

2) The value of a, called the significance level, is defined. This value represents the probability of rejecting the null hypothesis when it is true. In this study, a=0.05 is used.

3) The ^-value is analysed and compared with the significance level a. The lower this value, the greater the evidence against the null hypothesis. If the p-value is less than or equal to a, the null hypothesis is rejected and the alternative hypothesis is accepted as true. These results obtained in the sample are also inferred for the population.

In addition to the test for proportions, the Confidence Interval was constructed, with a 95% confidence level for the proportions under study. This interval contains the true proportion with a probability of 95%.

CHAPTER 5

RESULTS

A total of 402 interviews were conducted with members of the nursing team - 73 nurses, 284 technicians and 45 nursing assistants. The answers, framed in a questionnaire with 18 questions, were tabulated and submitted to statistical analysis as described below.

5.1 PROFILE OF THE INTERVIEWEES

The profile of the interviewees was analysed using questions relating to their professional training, the care they take with patients' oral hygiene and other characteristics such as age, monthly salary and the type of establishment they work in.

The table below shows the descriptive summary for age.

TABLE 1 - Descriptive summary for the age of the interviewees.

	Minimum	Maximum	Average	Fashion
Age	19	64	34	35

The average age of the interviewees was 34. The minimum observed was 19, the maximum was 64 and the most frequent was 34.

The following graph shows the percentage of interviewees according to age group and gender.

Percentual dos entrevistados segundo faixa etária e gênero.

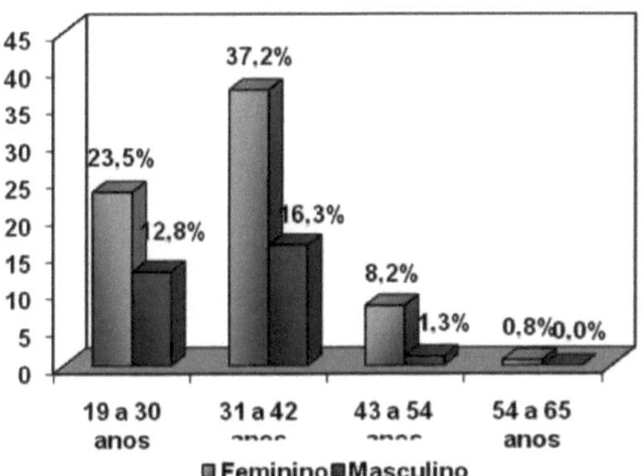

GRAPH 1 - Percentage of interviewees according to age group and gender.

Percentual dos entrevistados segundo categoria profissional e gênero.

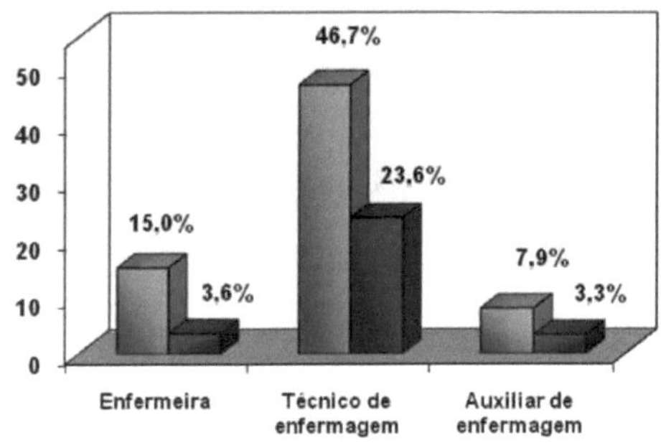

■ Feminino ■ Masculino

GRAPH 2 - Percentage of interviewees according to professional category and gender.

The graph above shows that the percentage of women is higher than the percentage of men in all three professional categories. The nursing technician category, in both genders, has the highest percentage compared to the other categories.

The interviews focused mainly on public and private hospitals. Several professionals pointed out that they work in more than one type of establishment, which is quite common. Other types of establishments were also included in the survey, such as private clinics, basic health units, institutions or nursing homes for the elderly, etc.

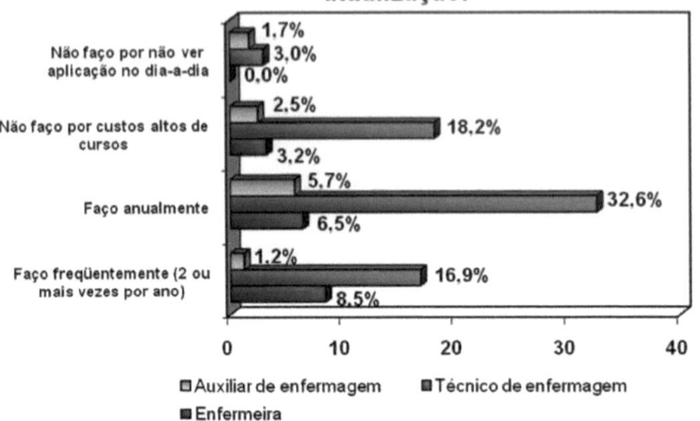

GRAPH 3 - Proportion of interviewees according to the frequency with which they attend refresher courses

The majority of those interviewed, in all three professional categories, say they take refresher courses every year.

5.2 ANALYSING THE INTERDISCIPLINARY RELATIONSHIP

We found that in all categories, the majority of professionals work in interdisciplinary teams, as shown in the table below.

TABLE 2 - Frequency and percentage of interviewees according to professional category and work in a multi/interdisciplinary team.

	Yes		No		Total	
	Frequency	%	Frequency	%	Frequency	%
Nurse	72	17,9	1	0,2	73	18,2
Nursing technician	277	68,9	7	1,7	284	70,6
Nursing assistant	45	H,2	0	o,o	45	11,2
Total	394	98,0	8	2,0	402	100,0

With regard to the presence of an effective dental surgeon in the interdisciplinary team, TABLE 3 shows that almost all of the interviewees replied that the teams they were part of did not have a dental surgeon. Furthermore, 86 per cent of those interviewed considered it necessary to have a dental surgeon on the team, who could act in cases where dentistry was involved, as shown in GRAPH 4.

TABLE 3- Frequency and percentage of interviewees according to the availability of a dental surgeon as a permanent member of the work team.

	Frequency	%
Yes	1	0,25
No	393	99,75
Total	394	100,00

roporção dos entrevistados segundo a necessidade de cirurgião dentista na equipe de trabalho.

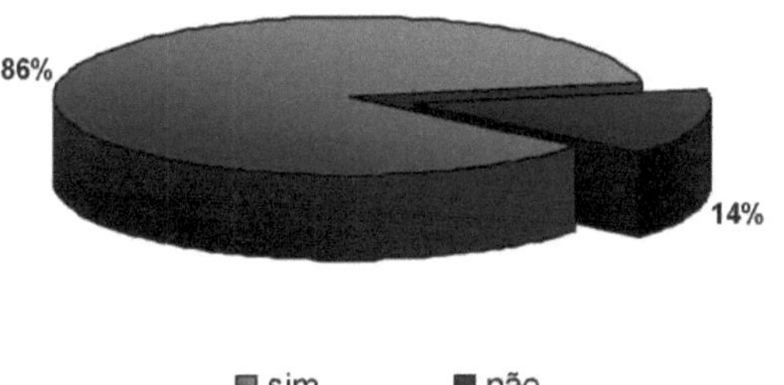

GRAPH 4 - Proportion of professionals with regard to the presence of a DS in interdisciplinary teams working in ICUs

With regard to the need for a DS to be present in interdisciplinary teams, the proportions comparison test was applied to test the following hypotheses:

Ho : The proportion (p) of respondents who consider it necessary to have a dental surgeon on staff is equal to the proportion who don't (p =0.5).

HI**:** The proportion (p) of those who consider the presence of a dental surgeon necessary is higher (p >0.5).

Result: p-value = 0.000.

Conclusion: As the p-value**: 0.000**, obtained in the test, is lower than the significance level of 0.05, the null hypothesis is rejected, i.e. the proportion of interviewees who consider the presence of a dental surgeon in the team to be necessary is higher than the proportion who do not.

Confidence interval for the proportion of those who consider it necessary to have a dental surgeon on the team: CI=**[85.0% ; 87.4%].**

With regard to knowledge of the oral health/general health relationship, 99 per cent of those interviewed agreed with the statement that an infection in the mouth can damage the health of the rest of the body (TABLE 4). In addition, 99.2% of respondents believe that mouth hygiene is important during a hospital stay (TABLE 5).

TABLE 4 - Frequency and percentage of professionals according to professional category and agreement with the statement that oral infection can jeopardise the health of the rest of the body.

	Yes	No	Total

	Frequency	%	Frequency	%	Frequency	%
Nurse	72	18,0	0	0	72	18,0
Nursing technician	279	69,8	4	1	283	70,8
Nursing assistant	45	H,3	0	0	45	11,3
Total	396	99,0	4	1	400	100,0

TABLE 5 - Frequency and percentage of interviewees according to professional category and knowledge that mouth hygiene is important during hospital stays.

	Yes		No		Total	
	Frequency	%	Frequency	%	Frequency	%
Nurse	70	17,5	1	0,3	71	17,8
Nursing technician	281	70,4	2	0,5	283	70,9
Nursing assistant	45	H,3	0	0,0	45	11,3
Total	396	99,2	3	0,8	399	100,0

5.3 ANALYSIS OF ORAL HEALTH KNOWLEDGE

List of the oral care you provide and/or advise your patients on

We can see that the examination of the oral cavity and/or advice to seek out a dental professional to carry it out is not carried out, according to the answers given by 37 per cent of the professionals. For one group, representing approximately 63 per cent of those interviewed, oral examination and/or guidance is carried out (GRAPH 5).

Proporção dos entrevistados que realizam/orientam seus pacientes segundo "exame da cavidade bucal".

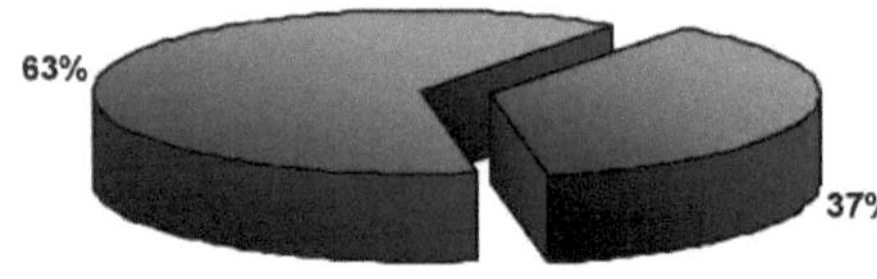

realiza/orienta
não realiza/orienta

GRAPH 5 - Proportion of interviewees who carry out and/or guide their patients according to oral cavity examination

Proporção dos entrevistados que realizam/orientam seus pacientes segundo "interrupção do uso de próteses".

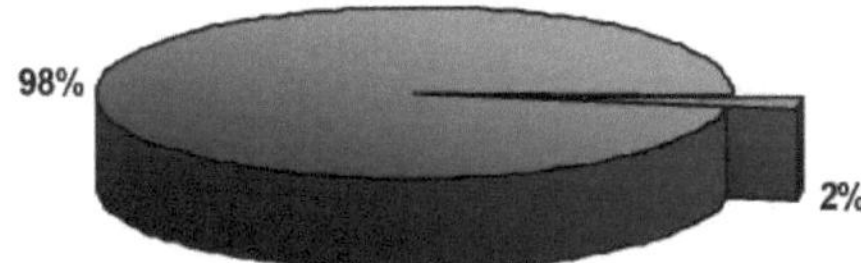

realiza/orienta
não realiza/orienta

GRAPH 6 - Proportion of interviewees who perform and/or guide their patients according to "discontinuation of prosthesis use"

Proporção dos entrevistados que realizam/orientam seus pacientes segundo "higienização com gaze ou bastão antiséptico".

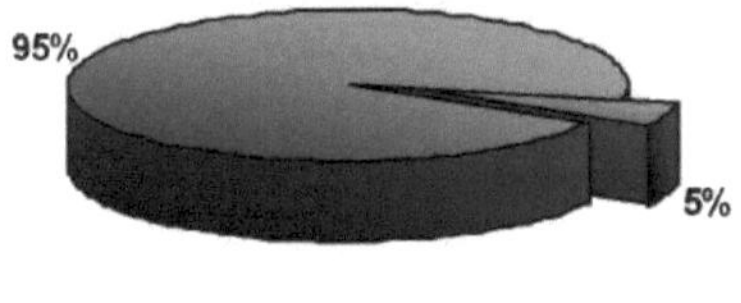

realiza/orienta
não realiza/orienta

GRAPH 7 - Proportion of interviewees who sanitise their patients with gauze or an antiseptic stick.

The professionals interviewed also answered questions about whether they carry out and guide their patients through the following procedures: normal tooth brushing; use of a bedside brushing tray; mouth rinses; hygienisation of dentures; and recommending the use of dentures in conscious patients. The results and statistical analyses obtained are shown in the following graphs:

Proporção dos entrevistados que realizam/orientam seus pacientes segundo "escovação dental normal".

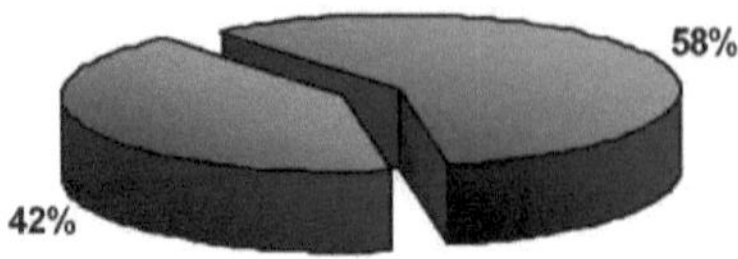

realiza/orienta
não realiza/orienta

GRAPH 8 - Proportion of interviewees who perform/guide their patients according to "normal tooth brushing"

Hypotheses:

Ho : The proportion (p) of interviewees who perform/guide their patients on normal tooth brushing is equal to the proportion who do not perform/guide. (p =0.5) H_1: The proportion (p) of those who perform/guide is lower. (p <0.5).

Result: p-value = 0.001.

Conclusion: As the p-value**: 0.001**, obtained in the test, is lower than the significance level of 0.05, we conclude that the proportion of interviewees who perform/guide their patients on normal tooth brushing is lower than the proportion who do not perform/guide. Confidence interval for the proportion of interviewees who perform/guide their patients in normal tooth brushing: CI=[**55.6%** ; **60.4%**].

Proporção dos entrevistados que realizam/orientam seus pacientes ͤgundo "uso de cuba para escovação no leito".

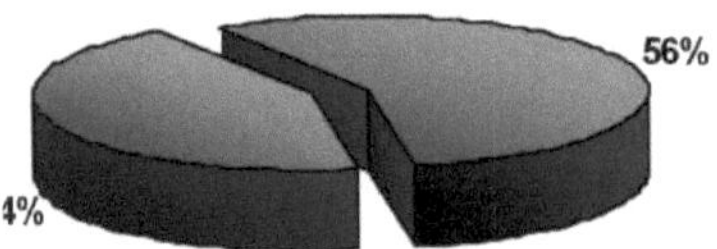

realiza/orienta
não realiza/orienta

GRAPH 9 - Proportion of interviewees who carry out/guide their patients according to "use of bedside brushing tub"

Hypotheses:

Ho: The proportion (p) of respondents who use a bedside brushing tray is equal to the proportion who don't (p =0.5).

H1**:** The proportion (p) of those who use is lower (p <0.5).

Result: p-value = 0.009.

Conclusion: As the p-value **is 0.009**, less than 0.05, the null hypothesis is rejected, i.e. the proportion of interviewees who use a bedside brush is lower than the proportion who do not.

Confidence interval for the proportion of interviewees who use **bedside** brushing**:** CI=**[41.4%** ; **46.4%]**.

Proporção dos entrevistados que realizam/orientam seus pacientes segundo "bochechos".

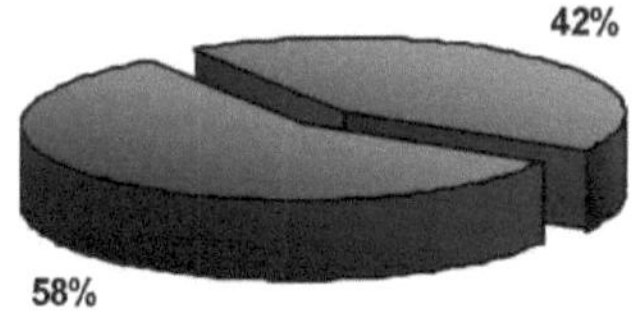

realiza/orienta
não realiza/orienta

GRAPH 10 - Proportion of interviewees who perform/guide their patients according to "mouthwashes"

Ho: The proportion (p) of respondents who perform/guide their patients with regard to mouthwashes is equal to the proportion who don't (p =0.5).

H1**:** The proportion (p) of those who perform/guide is different from the proportion of those who do not perform/guide (p #0.5)

Result: *p-value* = 0.002.

Conclusion: As the p-value is **0.002**, we accept the hypothesis that the proportion of interviewees who perform/guide mouthwashes is different from the proportion who do not.

Confidence interval for the proportion of interviewees who perform/guide their patients with regard to mouthwashes: IC=**[55.4% ; 60.2%]**.

This range shows proportions greater than 50 per cent, indicating that the proportion of those who perform/orient their patients with regard to mouthwashes is greater than the proportion who do not perform/orient.

Proporção dos entrevistados que realizam/orientam seus pacientes segundo "higienização das próteses".

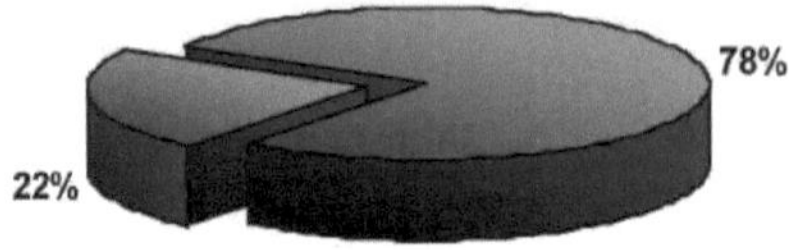

realiza/orienta
não realiza/orienta

GRAPH 11 - Proportion of interviewees who perform/orient their patients according to "hygiene of dentures"

Ho: The proportion (p) of interviewees who perform/guide their patients on denture hygiene is equal to the proportion who do not perform/guide. ($p = 0.5$) **H1:** The proportion (p) of those who perform/guide is lower. ($p < 0.5$) **Result:** p-value = 0.000.

Conclusion: As the p-value obtained in the test is **0.000,** the hypothesis is accepted that the proportion of interviewees who carry out/guide their patients on prosthesis hygiene is lower than the proportion who do not.

Confidence interval for the proportion of interviewees who carry out/guide their patients on prosthesis hygiene: CI=**[20.6% ; 23.9%]**.

Proporção dos entrevistados segundo "recomendação de uso de próteses em pacientes conscientes".

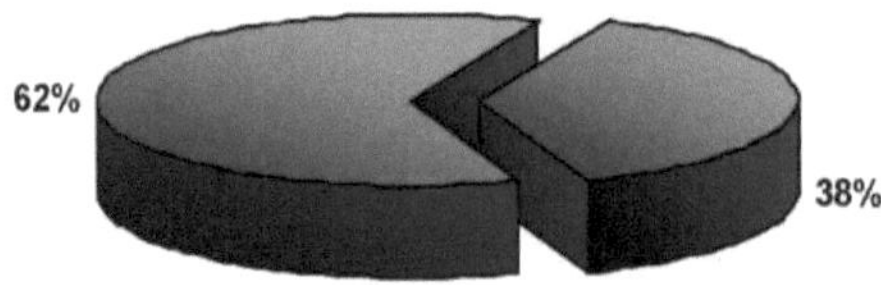

não utilizar   utilizar

GRAPH 12 - Proportion of interviewees according to the recommendation to use prostheses in conscious patients

Ho: The proportion (p) of respondents who do not recommend the use of prostheses in conscious patients is equal to the proportion who do (p =0.5).

HI**:** The proportion (p) of those who do not recommend is higher (p >0.5).

Result: p-value = 0.000.

Conclusion: As the p-value of **0.000** obtained in the test is lower than the significance level of 0.05, the hypothesis is accepted that the proportion of interviewees who do not recommend the use of prostheses in conscious patients is higher than the proportion who do.

Confidence interval for the proportion of respondents who do not recommend the use of prostheses in conscious patients: **IC=[59.9% ; 64.5%].**

When the interviewees were asked, in an open question, to name the most commonly used brand of mouthwash, we obtained a 100.00% response rate for Cepacol.

Xerostomia has been a growing problem in the hospital patient population due to the use of drugs with this side effect, therapies for oncological treatment, some autoimmune disorders or diabetes. Some products, available on the market in the form of gels, sprays, toothpastes, mouthwashes and even chewing gum, act on the oral tissues to soften the effects of dry mouth. These resources, however, are little publicised in the nursing profession: approximately 90% of those interviewed said they had never heard of these products and, with regard to their use in hospitals, none of them reported any isolated experience of coming into contact with these resources.

Some products have an effect on denture fixation in patients with dry mouth. In this case, the characteristics of the dentures must be taken into account, such as retention, marginal sealing, presence of saliva, etc. With regard to denture fixatives, approximately 25 per cent of professionals are familiar with them and, in the hospital, their use was not reported.

In the interdental areas, toothpicks can be used as a substitute for dental floss. They should be made of soft wood and triangular in shape to adapt to this area. There is still a lack of studies to prove their efficiency and control the harm that these instruments can cause. The toothpick format recommended is different from the model found in one of the hospitals and, according to the results obtained in the interviews, almost 100% of those interviewed are familiar with this method.

When assessing the knowledge of nursing professionals on various dental topics, approximately 30 per cent of those interviewed said they knew about tooth brushing techniques. Approximately 76% said they recognised the normal aspects of the oral cavity and when it came to the most common diseases of the oral cavity, such as dental caries, gingivitis, periodontitis and candidiasis, 29% were unaware. Among those interviewed, 30% thought they knew about cleaning dentures and discontinuing their use, and 29% said they knew about mucosal hygiene. As for cleaning the tongue, approximately 40 per cent said they were familiar with the subject and affirmed their ability to advise patients if asked.

Only 21.66 per cent of the target population is instructed to visit the dentist regularly and to prevent oral cancer. We found that 78.34% of the professionals recognised that they do not instruct patients to go to the dentist, nor do they give advice on oral cancer prevention.

The question was asked as to whether the members of the nursing team had received specific training on oral hygiene during their professional training. The graph below shows that approximately 42 per cent of the professionals had some knowledge of the subject.

Proporção dos entrevistados segundo realização de treinamentos específicos para a higiene da boca durante sua formação profissional.

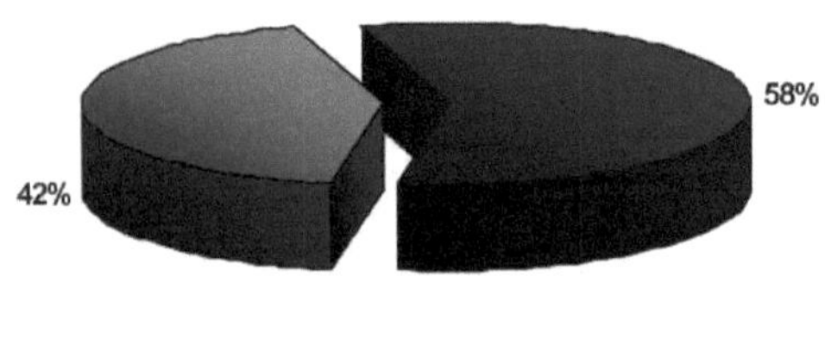

■ sim ■ não

GRAPH 13 - Proportion of interviewees according to specific training in oral hygiene during their professional training

Ho: The proportion (p) of interviewees who underwent specific training in oral hygiene during their professional training is equal to the proportion who did not.

(p=0.5)

H1: The proportion (p) of those who have done it is lower (p <0.5).

Result: p-value = 0.001.

Conclusion: With a p-value of **0.001**, we accept the hypothesis that the proportion of those who underwent specific training during their professional training is lower than the proportion who did not.

Confidence interval for the proportion of interviewees who received specific training in oral hygiene during their professional training: **CI=[40.0% ; 44.8%].**

However, in all the categories we found that 74 per cent of the sample rated the effectiveness of the training provided as insufficient (GRAPH 14).

Proporção de entrevistados segundo classificação dos treinamentos para higiene da boca, realizados durante sua formação profissional.

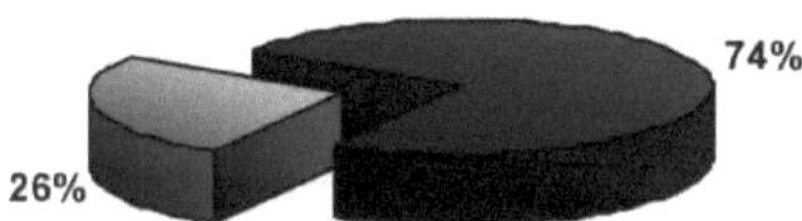

Suficientes ■ Insuficientes

GRAPH 14 - Proportion of interviewees according to the classification of oral hygiene training received during their professional training.

Ho: The proportion (p) of respondents who consider specific training in oral hygiene, carried out during their professional training, to be sufficient to care for patients' oral problems is equal to the proportion who do not. (p =0.5) H_1**:** The proportion (p) of those who have done so is lower. (p <0.5).

Result: p-value = 0.000.

Conclusion: With a p-value of **0.000**, the hypothesis is accepted that the proportion of those who consider the training they received during their professional training to be sufficient to look after patients' oral health is lower than the proportion who do not.

Confidence interval for the proportion of respondents who consider the specific oral hygiene training they received during their professional training to be sufficient to deal with patients' oral problems:

IC=[23.1% ; 28.9]

When asked if they would like to know more about oral health and the application of this knowledge to the patients they see, 98.5 per cent were almost unanimous in their interest in this subject.

CHAPTER 6

DISCUSSION

According to the literature, toothbrushes are the oral care tool of choice selected by nurses (KITE and PEARSON, 1995; HARRIS, 1980). In addition, there is extensive evidence linking the use of toothbrushes to effective control of plaque and its complications. Toothbrushes are the utensils of choice for oral care. Toothbrushing, combined with fluoride toothpastes, is recommended for almost all patients (JENKINS, 1989; HAYES and JONES, 1995). Only a minority of intubated patients with severe ulcerations or haemorrhages on the oral mucosa should not have their teeth brushed. Intubated edentulous patients should have their tongue brushed to help keep the mucosa healthy. Dentures should be properly sanitised and ready for use immediately after disintubation (ERICKSON, 1997). To facilitate use in intubated patients, small-headed brushes can be effective (HAYES and JONES, 1995). Special autoclaves for toothbrushes and electric toothbrushes are other pieces of equipment that are available, but have not yet been tested on intubated patients (ABIDIA, 2007). When brushing is not possible, foam sticks soaked in chlorhexidine can be effective in reducing plaque. Chlorhexidine is effective against gram-positive and gram-negative bacteria and fungi (HENNESSEY, 1973). Chlorhexidine also shows great affinity with the oral mucosa, tooth surfaces and saliva glycoproteins and has a bacteriostatic action lasting approximately twelve hours (SCANNAPIECO, 1998). Recently, 0.12% chlorhexidine solutions without alcohol in their composition have been developed and are considered as effective as those composed of 0.2% chlorhexidine, with alcohol being one of its other components and therefore indicated for use (VAN STRYDONCK et al., 2005). Foam sticks soaked in antimicrobial solutions are more effective for rinsing and moisturising the oral cavity when applied between brushings (JENKINS, 1989; BARNASON, 1998).

It has also been claimed that 0.9% saline solutions or water are just as effective as oral rinses (JENKINS, 1989; LIWU, 1990). Disposable cotton swabs are often used to clean and moisturise the mucous membranes and teeth of ICU patients. Examples of these utensils are lemon and glycerine swabs which initially stimulate saliva production but are acidic, causing irritation and decalcification of the teeth, so choosing less erosive products is of paramount importance (ADAMS, 1996; MEURMAN, 1996).

A protocol for oral care in ICUs is needed (FITCH et al., 1999). HAYES and JONES (1995) formatted a protocol called the "Examination Model" with information on signs and symptoms that should be noted in the patient's oral cavity by the nursing team at the time. Bleeding gums, redness, ulcerations, halitosis, among others, were suggested signs to be investigated by the professional in charge using the protocol.

Oral hygiene in ICUs is considered a routine nursing procedure whose aim is to keep the patient's oral cavity healthy (KITE and PEARSON, 1995; PRITCHARD and DAVID, 1988; BERRY, 2006) reported that oral care is necessary to maintain cleanliness, prevent infections/stomatitis, keep the oral mucosa moist and promote patient comfort.

Generally, the nursing team is not adequately trained in the treatment of the ICU patient's oral cavity, and protocols that serve as a guide to information are not available in the workplace (FITCH et al. 1999; BERRY,2006). It has been recommended that dental professionals be integrated into nursing training programmes with the aim of improving the knowledge and practical skills of the team, promoting better quality of care.

Fitch et al. (1999) recommended the implementation of an oral care protocol for nursing staff on examination techniques and oral hygiene.

Some solutions and equipment used by nurses for mouth treatment are not suitable (KITE and PEARSON, 1995). Hydrogen peroxide and sodium bicarbonate remove plaque, but if they are not handled with caution, they can cause superficial burns. In one study using hydrogen peroxide, significant changes to the mucosa were reported. Swabs, commonly used in the oral hygiene of dependent patients, are effective at stimulating mucosal tissues, but ineffective at removing plaque.

The frequency of oral care for intubated patients is an area of controversy. Jenkins (1989) suggested that the frequency of oral hygiene should vary, depending on the classification patients received in terms of the risk of obtaining oral pathologies, while Roth and Creason (1986) recommended intervals of two to four hours, depending on the patient's condition. The hygiene protocol suggested by Barnason (1998) established that brushing should be carried out every twelve hours and moisturising the mouth at least every two hours while the patient remained intubated. The author states that more in-depth research on the subject is still needed.

This study contributes to the realisation that dentistry plays an important role in maintaining and recovering the oral health of individuals hospitalised in intensive care units and, consequently, the general health of the human being. It is important that other health professionals have adequate knowledge of dentistry and are also aware of the most prevalent physiological and pathological oral alterations in hospitalised individuals.

It is known that dental problems affecting the oral cavity are more prevalent in bedridden people, mainly due to structural changes in the mucosa, decreased salivary flow, reduced immunological factors, among others. In this sense, in agreement with Abdida (2007), hospitalised patients require greater care from nurses when it comes to oral hygiene, always with a view to restoring general health as soon as possible.

This study proved the theory that defines the nursing team as a team of professionals who must be prepared to take on these new roles (POTTER and PERRY, 1999; REZENDE, 2005; BRUNETTI; MONTENEGRO, 2003). Virginia Henderson, in 1966, already described the essential role of the nurse:

> (...) to assist the individual, whether sick or healthy, in carrying out those activities that contribute to his health or recovery (or his peaceful death), which he would carry out alone if he had the necessary strength, will or knowledge. And to do so in such a way as to help them achieve independence as quickly as possible.

As it is a practice-orientated discipline, nursing concepts have evolved over time (GERMANO, 1993) and today the activities carried out by these professionals have been established in nursing codes, including new fields of activity, always reflecting a vision of man as a complete biopsychosocial being.

In recent decades, interviews have shown that the participation of these professionals has increased significantly, both in absolute numbers and in terms of the number of professionals per inhabitant (DU GAS, 1984; PUPULIM and SAWADA, 2002). This has led to an increase in the demand for administrative nursing jobs and we also realise the importance of training nursing assistants who already work in this area (Ministry of Health, 2001).

Specifically in Brazil, three categories of nursing are recognised: nurses, nursing technicians and nursing assistants. This profession is carried out by people who are legally qualified and registered with the Regional Nursing Councils (COREN).

Nurses are qualified by undergraduate courses at recognised institutions and are responsible for running institutional health units and heading up nursing services, organising and directing these services, as well as technical and auxiliary activities.

Nursing technicians carry out mid-level activities. They guide and monitor the work of assistants and take part in planning nursing care.

The assistant carries out medium-level activities of a repetitive nature, involving auxiliary nursing services under supervision and taking part in simple executions of treatment processes (BRASIL, 1986).

This dissertation looked at the three levels of nursing professionals. It was noted that nurses have a higher level of education than technicians and assistants, and are responsible for guiding the other members of the team.

For this reason, we conclude that the coinciding results obtained by the survey possibly indicate a predominance of standard nurse thinking. In this sense, we realise that the lack of knowledge in relation to dentistry covers all categories.

Based on the results obtained from the interviews, it can be seen that the vast majority of this research was applied to women, perhaps because this gender is more likely to follow the professions outlined in the questionnaire (Ministry of Health, 2001). Nursing is a mainly female profession in most countries of the world, although the participation of men has been increasing, but they still don't represent 2% of all nurses (DU GAS, 1984) (Ministry of Health, 2001).

In Brazil, the average age of nurses is 31, while in the United States it is 40 and in Canada it is 35. Not so long ago, the majority of nurses were young, unmarried women professionals, and nowadays the average age has increased as a trend indicating that nurses are staying in work for longer (DU GAS, 1984). In Brazil in particular, the higher education category of nursing is relatively new and nursing courses are becoming more common in universities, which may be related to the presence of younger professionals (Ministry of Health, 2001).

Like Rezende (2005) and Brunetti and Montenegro (2003), this study found that although nursing is a growing activity, for many of these professionals the labour market still offers unsatisfactory pay, a fact that forces many individuals to work in more than one establishment to supplement their monthly family income.

Currently, the places where nursing staff are most concentrated are hospitals and care homes for sick people. Few professionals carry out community activities in nursing homes, outpatient clinics and homes, but studies show that these are the future fields of care. The same conclusion was reached by Du Gas during a study carried out in 1984.

Another point for discussion is the fact that more than half of the professionals regularly update their knowledge, especially the nurses. However, this evaluation did not address the topics of the courses they usually attend or whether they deal with oral health issues, which could suggest that dentistry has carried out its activities at a distance from the other health professions. Thus, we can reflect on the question of whether dentistry and nursing follow different paths in patient care.

Contrary to the above statement, we realise that the principles of an interdisciplinary team have been highly disseminated nowadays, especially when it comes to ICU care (GENCO and GROSSI, 1998). During the interviews, there were frequent doubts about the meaning of an interdisciplinary or multidisciplinary team. They thought about the appropriate terminology, saying that multidisciplinary would be related to the numerous branches of knowledge that provide health care, while the concept of interdisciplinarity transcends this idea, referring to disciplinary reciprocity, considering situations common to two or more disciplines and the exchange of knowledge between members of the health team.

To add to the discussion, it's worth noting that the hospitals we visited employ professionals from various fields of expertise, including administrative staff in different categories, hospital cleaners and maintenance service providers and food service providers. Some activities in certain hospitals are outsourced.

As far as direct patient care is concerned, most establishments are staffed by doctors in various specialities, nurses, technicians and nursing assistants. Other professionals are found less frequently, such as physiotherapists, nutritionists and psychologists. Some hospitals received patients who had undergone surgical procedures performed by dentists, in this case specialists in oral and maxillofacial surgery and traumatology (MBFMT).

Thus, we realised that the interdisciplinary teams that many interviewees claimed to be part of don't actually exist if we compare the principles that govern these teams (REZENDE, 2005). We have professionals from different fields of knowledge in the health area, but the exchange between them is inexpressive or even non-existent (SOUZA et al., 2001). The dialogue that is so important for solving problems presented by patients has still not managed to overcome the obsolete hierarchies of our society.

Based on the questioning of the presence of an effective dental surgeon, who would be directly responsible for cases involving dentistry, we consider, firstly, that hospitals should review their concepts of interdisciplinary teams, so that the entry of a dental surgeon into the hospital environment can be justified in accordance with (IACOPINO, 1997; REYNOLDS, 1997; MARTINS FILHO e SANTOS, 2005).

Among those interviewed, the unanimous response was that the hospitals they were part of did not have a dental surgeon, and possibly they were not even aware of the work of dentists specialising in CTBMF who, in fact, carry out procedures in operating theatres and, at other times, keep patients in hospital.

Thus, none of the institutions visited had dentists responsible for oral health care in intensive care units. We can see from the statistical analysis of this study that even though their attention is not focused on prevention and oral hygiene care, it supports the statement by Puricelli and Wells (1996) when they emphasise that dental surgeons specialising in CTBMF can contribute, to a certain extent, to the knowledge of nurses.

The presence of a dental surgeon in hospital teams is necessary for 86% of those interviewed, who recognise that the dentist could act in cases where there is dental involvement. The literature on dentistry in interdisciplinary practice, specifically in ICUs, is recent in Brazil, with few mentions of dentists working in this sector before the 1990s, in contradiction to many other countries. However, due to the growth in the number of scientific studies in the field of dentistry relating oral alterations to many other organic alterations, there has been a concomitant increase in interest in so-called hospital dentistry.

From this perspective, knowledge about the relationship between oral health and general health was addressed in this study with a high level of agreement. The interviewees recognise that oral health is important for the general health of individuals and all agree on the importance of oral hygiene for patients hospitalised in ICUs (LOGAN et al. 1991; BLANK et al. 1996; GRAP, 2003; BINKLEY et al. 2004). Despite this, there is no interest in hiring dentists to work in this sector.

During visits to ICUs, it was observed that some patients may not need mechanical ventilation and may be able to carry out their own basic hygiene care, requiring help from nursing staff (TIMBY, 2001; ALEXANDRE and BRITO, 2000). It is therefore important to assess patients' degree of independence, as self-care should be stimulated and patient independence encouraged, not in order to reduce nursing obligations, but to stimulate patient recovery (ATKINSON and MURRAY, 1989).

Atkinson and Murray (1989) emphasise checking the use of prostheses at the time of hospitalisation and identifying those that are not being used. In these cases, it is recommended that they be kept in labelled cups. The data obtained in this study showed that approximately 100 per cent of patients do not use their prostheses, even if they do not require mechanical ventilation. In the majority of cases, it was found that the prostheses were handed over to the family or carers at the time of admission to these units, contrary to Erickson, 1997; Potter and Perry, 1999; Lauria et al., 2003, when they drew attention to the importance of using these utensils whenever possible in the hospital environment to prevent a variety of alterations that can be caused, such as changes to the mucosa, a reduction in the vertical dimension of occlusion and resorption of alveolar bone.

According to Amâncio and Cavalcante (1975) and Erickson (1997), patients should have proper oral hygiene even when they have no teeth. The authors suggest massages to strengthen the gums and rinsing the dentures to remove food debris that can injure and bother the patient. They also add that it is the nurse's responsibility to observe the patient's oral state, checking whether they wear dentures, whether they can feed themselves and whether they can chew. However, it was observed that no differentiated procedures are administered to partially or totally edentulous patients in the ICUs selected for this study.

In line with these thoughts, in our study we questioned the frequency with which the oral cavity was examined and observed a deficiency in carrying out the examination, which can be considered essential care and which we suggest should be included in the patient's medical records. The table below is a suggestion for a dental chart with simplified data on the patient's oral condition.

TABLE 6 - Suggested dental form with simplified data on the patient's oral condition

Use of removable full or partial dentures (dentures, bridges...)	□ Superior	□ Lower
Use of Mechanical Ventilation	□ Yes	□ No
Needs sanitising in bed	□ Yes	□ No
Changes in the oral mucosa	□ Yes	□ No
Inflammation or bleeding in the mouth	□ Yes	□ No
Patient's condition:	Comments:	

When examining an ICU patient, it is important to pay special attention to the supporting soft tissues and any alterations to the normal aspects of the mucous membranes. The absence of this control can lead to damage to the supporting tissues, muscles, TMJ, dental elements and the development of pathologies (stomatitis, gingivitis, hyperplasia, precancerous and malignant lesions) not being noticed and worsening the patient's state of health.

Guidance on oral care should be tailored to the patient's motor skills and cognitive ability. In this way, the preventive purposes must be understood by the patient and their support group (family members and/or nursing staff), according to (BRUNETTI & MONTENEGRO, 2003).

Often, physical or mental causes prevent satisfactory oral hygiene, requiring the assistance of someone who is properly trained. A guide that can also be suggested to nursing staff on the relationship between the need for proper oral hygiene procedures and different levels of patient dependency can be found in the table below:

TABLE 7 - Guidance suggested to nursing staff on the relationship between the need for adequate oral hygiene procedures and different levels of patient dependency

<table>
<tr><th colspan="3">Level of Dependence X Oral Hygiene</th></tr>
<tr><td>PATIENT INDEPENDENT</td><td>Patient who can walk</td><td>Go to a sink and wash yourself
Encourage and guide correct techniques</td></tr>
<tr><td rowspan="2">PARTIALLY DEPENDENT PATIENT</td><td>Patients who cannot travel</td><td>Provide a hygiene tub at the bedside</td></tr>
<tr><td>Patients with motor difficulties</td><td>Auxiliary features such as brushes with adapted handles, electric brushes...</td></tr>
<tr><td rowspan="2">DEPENDENT PATIENT</td><td>Patients with motor impairments</td><td>Hygiene performed by a carer or nursing staff with ordinary brushes or electric brushes</td></tr>
<tr><td>Intubated patient</td><td>Brushing and hygiene with gauze and 0.12% chlorhexidine antiseptic</td></tr>
</table>

Erickson (1997); Ziviani and Cruz (2006); Abidia (2007); Cutler and Davis (2005); Binkley et al. (2004); Wall et al. (2001) and Fitch et al. (1999) emphasised the prevention and promotion of oral health in ICUs through protocols designed according to the individual needs of ICU patients, recommending the mechanical removal of plaque in dentate individuals using correctly indicated toothbrushes. However, none of the teams observed followed any kind of individual oral hygiene protocol. The same procedure was carried out for all patients. Toothbrushes were rarely used by the individuals themselves, who were totally independent of special care, without guidance or encouragement from members of the team assisting them.

According to the aforementioned authors, chlorhexidine-containing agents are strategic for preventing caries, gingivitis and abscesses, and are recommended depending on the risk of developing such pathologies or when effective hygiene skills are compromised. Preventive oral cavity examinations are therefore recommended as a regular practice for hospitalised patients. Emphasising the importance of this care, this study sought to assess the oral hygiene resources that nursing staff know and use in their work environment and we realised from the results that little is known about plaque control methods and other resources for oral hygiene and maintaining the oral health of ICU patients.

The resources available in the hospitals visited can be considered scarce and the activities carried out need to be reviewed, which represents a difficulty in maintaining oral health and the impossibility of controlling oral infections that have already set in.

All the hospitals visited only have one type of mouthwash, and in all the institutions the brand used is Cepacol, which is an ineffective product. There were few establishments that provided their independent or partially dependent patients with oral hygiene materials. Most of the time, it was noted that the use of oral hygiene instruments depended on their own resources; when possible, the family was assigned to bring them from home. The oral hygiene kit provided to patients included only a child's toothbrush and a mouthwash.

Based on our research, it was possible to see that the nursing team responsible for the hygiene care of hospitalised patients has received little information about the plaque control methods responsible for the origin of the main oral pathologies and that they are also unaware of various oral hygiene resources that could be used in the hospital environment with significant improvements in the maintenance and recovery of the oral health of these individuals (LOGAN et al. 1991; BLANK, et al. 1996; GRAP et al., 2003; CUTLER and DAVIS, 2005; FITCH et al., 1999 and BERRY, 2006).

As for the frequency with which specific oral hygiene care is carried out, the opinions found by different authors (Jenkins, 1989; Roth and Creason, 1986; Barnason et al., 1998) vary. Brushing using a toothbrush and toothpaste should be advocated as essential basic care, so that it can be extended to all patients who need to receive this type of attention. We observed that oral hygiene procedures were only carried out twice a day in the ICUs chosen for our study, coinciding with bath time just before the start of the interval for family and carer visits.

Macedo and Lacaz Netto (1980) state that the best prevention is the mechanical removal of plaque through brushing, flossing and other means of hygiene. Various tooth brushing techniques are described in the literature and, if we compare the effect of tooth cleaning, no method is superior to another, as described by Lindhe and Karring (1999). These authors state that the willingness and ability of the patient, as well as the results obtained, regardless of the brushing technique used, are more important factors than the selection of the toothbrushing method. In 100% of the ICUs visited, the only oral hygiene technique used by the nursing staff was the use of sticks wrapped in gauze soaked in Cepacol.

As for manual toothbrushes, Galvão Filho (2004) reports that the existence of the toothbrush is estimated at 300 years. This instrument comes in a variety of shapes, thicknesses, consistencies and sizes. Several authors recommend brushes with soft bristles of equal height, rounded tips and small size (MACEDO and LACAZ NETTO, 1980). Lindhe and Karring (1999) state that the ideal toothbrush is one that can remove food debris well, performing its function correctly. In this study, we realised that this valuable resource could be better used in the hospital environment by increasing its use and the number of daily brushings.

Toothpaste or toothpastes used in combination with toothbrushes are one of the most effective means of controlling bacterial plaque (LASCALA, 1997). In addition to facilitating its removal, these agents have therapeutic and prophylactic purposes and may contain fluorides, antiseptics, enzymes and other substances (LINDHE and KARRING, 1999).

Toothbrushes, toothpaste and dental floss could be provided by the hospital so that tooth brushing is not jeopardised by the patient having to bring these resources from home.

Cylindrical or conical interdental brushes are prescribed for cleaning interdental spaces, when the space is wider or for people with fixed prostheses. Floss threaders are alternatives for cleaning fixed prostheses as they make it easier to floss the areas close to the gums, as shown by the aforementioned authors.

In the institutions covered by this research, however, we see that a large part of the nursing team is unaware of the existence of these resources, and their use in the hospital environment should be expanded.

Independent patients can perform their own oral hygiene using the bathroom sink. Bedridden patients, however, must perform this care in bed using a metal tub for emesis, and oral hygiene resources should be provided by the institution (TIMBY, 2001).

One resource widely used in the hospitals we visited is wooden sticks wrapped in gauze and soaked in antiseptics, especially Cepacol. There are few bibliographical references justifying the use of this solution, which is indicated for dependent or unconscious patients when hygiene with a toothbrush is impossible (ALEXANDRE and BRITO, 2000). However, in our research, such care is quite significant, especially in terms of the frequency with which it is carried out, and it is found to be the only oral hygiene care used by professionals. From this perspective, toothpicks, as stated by the authors Rezende, 2005; Brunetti and Montenegro, 2003, should have a restricted indication. Thus, it can be suggested that when the patient is unable to use toothbrushes, even small ones, hygiene should be carried out with the stick wrapped in gauze soaked in 0.12% chlorhexidine solution, a procedure defined as effective and long-lasting in reducing plaque formed by gram-positive and gram-negative bacteria, as well as having a great affinity with the oral mucosa, tooth surfaces and saliva glycoproteins (HAYES and JONES, 1995; HENNESSEY, 1973 and VAN STRYDONCK et al., 2005)

Our research recognised that, in fact, brush hygiene for totally or partially dependent patients requires greater skills and is more time-consuming. This seems to be one of the reasons for the application of care in the hospitals we visited. It is recommended that the care provided in the hospital be reviewed for the benefit of the patients admitted.

According to the Regional Nursing Council of the state of Pará (COREN), by 2007, 17,037 nursing professionals were registered in the city of Belém, divided into three professional categories. There were 2,507 registered nurses, 7,798 nursing technicians and 6,732 nursing assistants (table below), with no further details on the places and sectors they were working in at the time of the consultation. According to COREN, until 2007 there were only two registered nurses with a postgraduate qualification in intensive care units. For this reason, it was not possible to statistically correlate the professionals who had actually acquired postgraduate qualifications to work in ICUs with those who were interviewed during the survey.

TABLE 8 - Number of professionals registered with COREN in 2007

PROFESSIONAL CATEGORY	BELÉM
NURSES	2.507
NURSING TECHNICIANS	7.798
NURSING ASSISTANTS	6.732
SOURCE: COREN-PA	

By answering the questionnaire, 73 nurses, 284 nursing technicians and 45 nursing assistants agreed to take part in this study, totalling 402 professionals who were working in twenty-three intensive care units in the city of Belém, state of Pará.

It was decided to select hospitals that had at least eight beds available for adult patients in their ICUs. In this way, it was possible to approach the largest and most important hospitals and institutions in operation in the city where, consequently, most of the population is cared for. Smaller hospitals and private clinics, with an intensive care unit that mostly had one or two beds available, were not selected for the study in question. It was agreed that it would be very difficult to visit and get acceptance from all these smaller institutions, which would compromise the results obtained. Military hospitals were also visited by the researcher, but it was noted that in each of them there were only four beds available in an intensive care unit. Still on the smaller institutions, it was noted that their ICUs were managed by teams made up of a doctor and a nurse.

It was decided that if any of the interviewees worked in two different institutions on different shifts, they would be interviewed twice, so that there would be uniformity in the total number of members of each participating team. Although rare, there were records of interviewees not answering all the questions in some questionnaires of their own volition, a fact that was respected by the interviewer.

The strategy of using a single interviewer was adopted to avoid calibration errors between different interviewers (PERES, TRAEBERT & MARCENES, 2001).

The personal interview had great advantages in terms of direct contact with the interviewees. The use of a questionnaire formulated with closed questions was advocated in order to obtain definite answers. In this way, data analysis became more objective and tabulation and statistical analysis were simplified (MONTENEGRO, 1993).

We therefore suggest that integration between health professionals should become a reality within hospitals and that knowledge, previously restricted to one health speciality, should be better disseminated among the professionals who make up the health team, with the greatest beneficiary being the patient, the reason for all biomedical efforts. The nursing bibliographical references reviewed point to mostly correct behaviours, requiring only adaptations to national realities.

CHAPTER 7

CONCLUSION

Based on the results obtained and the literature consulted, the following conclusions were reached:

- The oral hygiene care provided to patients hospitalised in intensive care units in the city of Belém is precarious and inconsistent;
- In order to maintain oral health at satisfactory levels, changes are needed in the care currently provided by nursing teams in hospitals;
- Nursing staff know little about the methods of plaque control responsible for the main oral pathologies and the various products that can be used for oral hygiene;
- The resources available in the hospitals visited are scarce and inappropriate, making it impossible to maintain oral health and making it difficult to control oral infections that have already set in;
- The team that carries out oral hygiene care, in general, has not received adequate training to carry it out, and so we suggest that nursing curricula be revised and that knowledge of preventive dentistry be better disseminated among this class of professionals;
- The presence of a dental surgeon is suggested as an attempt to solve the difficulties presented in maintaining oral health and treating oral diseases that affect the general health of individuals hospitalised in ICUs;
- Interdisciplinary care in ICUs should include the presence of dental surgeons who are integrated into the principles of the teams involved. The knowledge disseminated in the hospital environment would be useful even after discharge, with a view to achieving quality of life for these patients.

BIBLIOGRAPHICAL REFERENCES

ABIDIA, R. F. Oral care in the intensive care unit: A review. **J. Contemp. Dent. Pract.,** v. 8, n. 1, p. 76-82, Jan. 2007.

ABIDIA, R. F.; AL-FARAN, K. Oral care in the intensive and intermediate care units in Riyadh and Qateef. **Pak Oral Dental J.,** v. 24, n. 1, p. 87-94, 2004

ADAMS, R. Qualified nurses inadequate knowledge related to oral health, resulting in inadequate oral care of patients on medical wards. **J. Adv. Nurs.,** v. 24, n. 1, p. 552-60, Sep. 1996.

ALEXANDRE, N. M. C.; BRITO, E. **Basic nursing procedures**. São Paulo: Atheneu, 2000. p. 13-15.

ALLBRIGHT, A. Oral care for the cancer chemotherapy patients. **Nurs. Times**, v. 80, n. 21 , p. 40-

2, 1984

ARAI, K. et al.. Association between dental health behaviours, mental/physial function and self-feeding ability among the elderly: a cross-sectional survey. **Gerontology,** v.20, n. 2, p. 78-83, Dec. 2003.

ARAÚJO, D. L. et al. **The importance of the dental surgeon in the care of patients admitted to the intensive care unit.** Available at: <http://www.odontologia.com.br/imprimir.asp?id=686&idesp=1. Accessed on: 13 Nov. 2007.

ASHURST, S. Nursing care of the mechanically ventilated patient in ITC:1. **Br. J. Nurs.,** v. 6, n, 8, p. 47-454, 1997.

ATKINSON, L. D.; MURRAY, M. E. **Fundamentals of Nursing**. Rio de Janeiro: Guanabara Koogan, 1989. p. 243- 245.

BAGRAMIAN, R. A.; HELLER, R. P. Dental health assessment of a population of nursing home residents. **J. Gerontol**., v. 32, n. 2, p. 168-174, Feb.1977.

BARKVOLL, P. et al. Interaction between chlohexidine digluconate and sodium monofluorophosphate in vitro. **Eur J. Oral Scie**., v. 96, n. 1, p. 30-33, Feb. 1988.

BARNASON, S.; GRAHAM, J.; WILD, M. C. Comparison of two endotracheal tube securement techniques onunplanned extubation, oral mucosa, and facial skin integrity. **Heart Lung,** v. 27, n. 6, p. 409-417, 1998.

BASILIO, R. C.; LODUCCA, F. E.; HADDAD, P. C. Medical prophylaxis of endocarditis. Braz. **J. Infect. Dis.**, v. 8, n. 5, p. 340-7, Oct. 2004.

BENTLEY, D. W. Bacterial pneumonia in the eldery: clinical features, diagnosis, etiology, and treatment. **Gerontology**, v. 30, n. 5, p. 297-307, 1984.

BERRY, A. M.; DAVIDSON, P. M. Beyond comfort: Oral hygiene as a critical nursing activity in the intensive care unit. **Intensive Crit. Care Nurs**., v. 22, n, 6, p. 318-28, Dec. 2006.

BINKLEY, C. et al. Survey of oral care practices in US intensive care units. **Am. J. Infect. Control**, v. 32, n. 3, p. 161-9, 2004.

BLANK, L. W.; ARVIDSON-BUFANO, U. B.; YELLOWITZ J. A. The effect of nurses' background on performance of nursing home resident oral health assessments pre - and post- training. **Spec. Care Dentist,** v. 16, n. 2, p. 65-70, Mar./Apr. 1996.

BOYCE, J. M. et al. Nosocomial pneumonia in medicare patients. Hospital costs and reimbursement patterns under the prospective payment system. **Arch. Intern. Med.**, v. 151, n. 6, p. 1109-14, Jun. 1991.

BRAZIL. **Decree No. 94.406** of 8 June 1987, which regulates Law No. 7.498 of 25 June 1986, which provides for the practice of nursing and makes other provisions. Brasília, 1987.

BRAZIL. Ministry of Health. **Parameters for programming basic health actions.** February 2001.

BROOK, I. M.; FREEMAN, C.; SHEFFIELD, D. J. L. ARF increase - letters. **Brit. Dent. J.**, v. 193, n. 4, p. 182-3, Aug. 2002.

BRUNETTI, R. F.; MONTENEGRO F. L .B.; MANETA, C. E. Functions of the masticatory system: its importance in the digestive process in geriatrics. **Actualidades em Geriatria,** v, 3, n. 16, 6- 9, abr. 1998.

BRUNETTI, R. F.; MONTENEGRO, F. L. B. Odontogeriatria: A new option for work in the 21st century. In: CARDOSO, R. J. A.; MACHADO, M. E. L. **Dentistry / Prosthodontics / TMJ / Implantology / Pre-prosthetic surgery / Odontogeriatrics**. São Paulo: Artes Médicas, 2003. Chap. 20, p. 441-453.

BRUNNER, S. C. S.; SUDDARTH, B. G. B. **Treatise on medical-surgical nursing. Vol. I.** 7. ed. Rio de Janeiro: Guanabara Koogan, 1992. p. 3-43.

____. **Treatise on medical-surgical nursing. Vol II** 7. ed. Rio de Janeiro: Guanabara Koogan, 1992. p. 401-756.

CARDENOSA CENDRERO, J. A. et al. Role of different routes of tracheal colonisation in the development of pneumonia in patients receiving mechanical ventilation. **Chest,** v. 116, n. 2, p. 462-70, Aug. 1999.

CARRANZA, F. A. **Glickman:** Clinical Periodontics. 7. ed. Rio de Janeiro: Guanabara Koogan, 1992.

CARRILHO, C. **Risk of developing hospital pneumonia in the ICU of the HURNP in Londrina.** In: CONGRESSO BRASILEIRO DE CONTROLE DE INFECÇÃO E EPIDEMIOLOGIA HOSPITALAR, 5., 1998. Campos do Jordão Proceedings..., 1998.

CARVALHO FILHO, E. T.; PAPALÉO NETTO, M. **Geriatria:** Fundamentos, clínica e terapêutica. São Paulo: Atheneu, 2000. p. 9-29.

CASSOLATO, S. F.; TURNBULL, R. S. **Gerontology**, v. 20, n. 2, p. 64-77, dec. 2003. Available at www.odontologia.com.br accessed in February 2004.

CLARK. D. C.; GUEST, J. L. The effectiveness of three different strengths of chlorhexidine mouthrinse. **J. Can. Dent. Assoc.,** v. 60, n. 8, p. 711-714, Aug. 1994.
LATIN AMERICAN CONSENSUS ON PNEUMONIA IN HOSPITALISED ADULT PATIENTS. San Juan, Puerto Rico, Jan. 1998.

LATIN AMERICAN CONSENSUS ON PNEUMONIA IN HOSPITALISED ADULT PATIENTS. San Juan, Puerto Rico, Jan. 1998.

COSTERTON, J. W. et al. Microbial biofilms. **Annu. Rev. Microbiol**., v. 49, p. 711-45, 1995.

CRAVEN, D. E.; STEGER, K. E.; BARBER, T. W. Preventing nosocomial pneumonia: state of the art and perspectives for the 1990s. **Am. J. Med.**, v. 91, n. 3b, 44S-53S, Sep. 1991.

CROWE, M.J.; COOKE, E.M. Review of case definitions for nosocomial infection- Towards a consensus. **J. Hosp. Infect**., London, n. 39, n. 1, p. 3-11, May. 1998.

CUTLER C. J.; DAVIS, N. Improving oral care in patients receiving mechanical ventilation. **Am. J. Crit. Care**, v. 14, n. 5, p. 389-394, Sep. 2005.

DAVID, C. M. N. Infection in the ICU. **Medicina, Ribeirão Preto**, v. 31, p. 337-348, jul.-set. 1998.

DAWES, C.; JENKINSG. V; TONGE, C. H. The nomenclature of the integuments of the enamel surface of the teeth. **Brit. Dent. J.**, v. 115, p. 65-68, 1973.

DAY, R. Mouth care in an intensive care unit: a review. **Intensive Crit. Care Nurs.**, v. 9, n. 4, p. 246-252, Dec. 1993.

DEPUYDT, P.; MYNY, D.; BLOT, S. Nosocomial pneumonia: aetiology, diagnosis and treatment. **Curr. Opin. Pulm. Med.,** v. 12, p. 192-197, 2006.

DERISO, A. J. et al. Chlorhexidine glugonate 0.12% oral rinse reduces the incidence of total nosocomial respiratory infection and nonprophylactic systemic antibiotic use in patients undergoing heart surgery. **Chest**, v. 109, n. 6, p. 1556-61, Jun. 1996.

DORO, G. M et al. "Hospital Dentistry" Project. **Revista da ABENO**, v. 6, p. 49-53, jan./jun. 2006

DU GAS, B. W. **Practical Nursing**. 4. ed. Rio de Janeiro: Guanabara Koogan, 1984, p. 29-409.

EPSTEIN, J. B. et al. "Benzydamine HCl for Prophylaxis of Radiation-Induced Oral Mucositis: Results From a Multicenter, Randomized, Double-Blind, Placebo-Controlled Clinical Trial," **Cancer,** v.92, n. 4, p. 875-85, 2001

ERICKSON, L. Oral health promotion and prevention for older adults. **Dent. Clin. of North Am.,** v. 41, n. 4, p. 727-750, Oct.1997.

FITCH, J. A. et al. Oral care in the adult intensive care unit. **Am. J. Crit. Care**, v. 8, n. 5, p. 314-8, Sep. 1999.

GADBURY-AMYOT, C. et al. Prioritisation of the National Dental Hygiene Research Agenda . **J. Dent.Hyg.**, v. 76, Issue 2, spring, 2002. p. 157-166.

GALVÃO FILHO, S. **Dicionário Odonto-Médico Inglês-Português.** 4. ed. São Paulo: Santos, 2004. 976p.

GASTINNE, H.; WOLFF, M.; DELATOUR, F. A controlled trial in intensive care units of selective decontamination of the digestive tract with nonabsorbable antibiotics. **N. Engl. J. Med.**, v. 326, p. 594-599, Feb.1992.

GENCO, R. J.; GROSSI, S. G.; Periodontal disease and diabetes mellitus: a two way relationship. Ann. Periodontol.1998; 3:51-61.

GEORGE, D. L. Nosocomial pneumonia. In: MAYHALL, C.G. **Hospital epidemiology and infection control. Baltimore**: Williams & Wilkins, 1996. Chap. 12, p. 175-95.

GERMANO, R. M. **Educação e ideologia da Enfermagem no Brasil.** 3. ed. São Paulo: Cortez, 1993.

GLASSMAN, P. et al. A preventive dentistry training programme for caretakes of persons with disabilities residing in communitu residential facilities. **Special Care in Dentistry**, v. 14, n. 4, p. 137-152, 1994.

GOLDIE, S. J. et al. Fungal peritonitis in a large chronic peritoneal dialysis population: a report of 55 episodes. **Am. J. Kidney Dis.,** v. 28, p. 86-91, 1996.

GRAP, M. et al. Oral care interventions in critical care: frequency and documentation. **Am. J. Crit. Care**, v. 12, n. 2, p. 113-8, 2003.

GROLLIER, G.; DORE P.; ROBERT R.; Antibody response to prevotella spp. In patients with ventilator-associated pneumonia. **Clin. Diag. Lab. Immunol.**, v. 3, n. 1, p. 61-65, Jan. 1996.

HALLET, N. Mouthcare. **Nurs. Mirror**, v. 159, v. 21, p. 31-3, Dec. 1984.

HANNEMAN, S. K.; GUSICK, G. M. Frequency of oral care and positioning of patients in critical care: a replication study. **Am. J. Crit. Care**, v. 14, p. 378-386, 2005.

HARRIS, N. G. Nutrition in ageing. In: MAHA, K.; ESCOTT-STUMP, S **Krause alimentos, nutrição e dietoterapia.**10. ed. São Paulo: Roca, 2002. Chap. 13, p. 276-295.

HAYES J.; JONES, C. A collaborative approach to oral care during critical illness. **Dent. Health,** v. 34, n. 3, p. 6-10, 1995.

HENDERSON, V. **The nature of nursing**. New York: Macmillan, 1966.

HILDEBRANDT, G. H. Effects of repeated treatment with sustained-release chlorhexidine mouth guards on salivary levels of Mutans Streptococci. **Caries Res.**, v. 30, n. 6, p. 445-453, 1996.

HUR, M. et al. Reduction of mouth malodour and volatile sulphur compounds in intensive care patients using an essential oil mouthwash. **Phytother Res**, v. 21, n. 7, p. 641-3, Jul. 2007.

IACOPINO, A. M. Understanding and treating aging patients. **Quintessence International**, v. 28, n. 9, p. 622-6, Sep. 1997.

JENKINS, D. A. Oral care in the ICU: an important nursing role. **Nurs. Stand**, v. 4, n. 7, p. 24-28,1989.

JONES H.; NEWTON J.; BOWER E. J. A survey of the oral care practices of intensive care nurses. Intensive care nurses. **Intensive Crit. Care. Nurs.**, v. 20, p. 69-76, 2004.

JORGE, A. O. C. **Microbiologia bucal**. 2. Ed. São Paulo: Santos, 1998. 122 p.

KAZOR, C. E. et al. Diversity of bacterial populations on the tongue dorsa of patients with halitosis and helthy patients. **J. Clin. Microbiol.**, v. 41, n. 2, p. 558-63, Feb. 2003.

KERVER, A. J. H.; ROMMES, J. H.; MEVISSEN-VERHAGE, E. A. E. Prevention of colonisation and infection in critically ill patients: a prospective randomized study. **Crit. Care Med.**, v. 16, p. 1087-1093, 1988.

KITE, K.; PEARSON, L. A Rationale for mouth care: the integration of theory with practice. **Intensive Crit. Care Nurs.,** v. 11, n. 2, p. 71-6, Apr. 1995.

KOEMAN, M. et al. Ventilator-associated pneumonia: recent issues on pathogenesis, prevention and diagnosis. **J. Hosp. Infect.**, v. 49, p. 155-62, 2001

KOIZUMI, M. S.; CIANCIARULLO, T. I. . Nursing assistance and nursing care. **Enfermagem em Novas Dimensoes**, São Paulo, v. 4, n. 1, p. 40-43, 1978.

KOMIYAMA, K.; TYNAN, J. J.; HABBICK, B. F. Pseudomonas aeruginosa in the oral cavity and sputum of patients with cystic fibrosis. **Oral Surg. Oral Med. Oral Pathol.**, v. 59, n. 6, p. 590-594, 1985.

LASCALA, N. T. **Prevenção na Clínica Odontológica:** promoção da saúde bucal. São Paulo: Artes Médicas, 1997. 314p.

LAURIA, R. A. et al. Evaluation of patients' knowledge about the use and care of complete dentures. **Pesqui. Odontol. Bras**. v. 17, supplement 2 (Proceedings of the 20th Annual Meeting of the SBPqO), 2003.

LAUS, A. M.; ANSELMI, M. L. Characterisation of patients admitted to the medical and surgical units of HCFMRP-USP, according to the degree of dependence on nursing care. **Rev. Latino-Am. Enfermagem**, v. 12, n. 4, jul./aug., 2004. Available in: <www.scielo.br/scielo.php?script=sci_arttext&pid=S0101-116920040004000010...> Accessed on: 28 Nov. 2004.

LEITE, J. A. **Analysis of the role of lingual scrapers in cleaning the oral cavity in elderly patients**. São Paulo, 2005.61f. Monograph (Specialisation in Odontogeriatrics) - ABENO.

LEITE, T. A. et al. Dental caries and sugar consumption in children attending a public day-care centre. **Rev. Odontol. Univ. São Paulo**, v. 13, n. 1, p. 13-18, jan./mar. 1999.

LEVISON, M. E. Pneumonia, including necrotising pulmonary infections (lung abscess). In: ISSELBACHER, K. J.; BRAUNWALD, E.; WILSON J. D. (eds). **Harrison's principles of internal medicine**. New York: McGrawn-Hill, 1994. p. 1184-1191.

LINDHE, J.; KARRING, T. **Treatise on clinical periodontics and oral implantology**. 3. ed. Rio de Janeiro: Guanabara Koogan, 1999.

LIWU A. Oral hygiene in intubated patients. **Aust. J. adv. Nurs.,** v. 7, n. 2, p. 4-7, 1990.

LOESCHE, W. J. et al. Dental findings in geriatric populations with diverse medical backgrounds. **Oral Surg Med Oral Pathol Oral Radiol Endod**, v. 80, n. 1, p. 43-54, Jul. 1995.

LOGAN, H. L.; ETTINGER, R.; McLERAN, H. Common misconceptions about oral health in the older adult: nursing practices. **Special Care in Dentistry**, v.11, n.6, p. 243-247, 1991.

LONGHURST, R. H.. A cross-sectional study of the oral health care instruction given to nurses during their basic training. **Br. Dent. J.**, v. 184, n. 9, p. 453-7, 1998.

MACEDO, N. L.; LACAZ NETTO, R. **Manual of oral hygiene**. São Paulo: Medisa, 1980, 72p.

MARSHALL, T. A. **Routine dental care is essential for adequate nutrition in the elderly.** Available at: www.medicenter.com Accessed on: 11 Dec. 2004.

MARTINO, M.D.V. Lower Respiratory Tract Infections. In: LEVY, C.E. et al. **Manual of clinical microbiology applied to hospital infection control**. São Paulo: APECIH, 1998. p. 3-10.

MARTINS FILHO, P. R. S.; SANTOS, T. S. Oral manifestations of diabetes mellitus. **Painel Online**. Available at: < www.aboprev.com.br> Accessed on: 8 Feb. 2005.

MCDONALD, A. M.; DIETSCHE, L.; LITSCHE, M. A. Retrospective study of nosocomial pneumonia at a long-term care facility. **Am. J. Infect. Cont.**, v. 20, p. 234-238, 1992.

MCKELLAR, P. P. Treatment of community acquiredpneumonias. **Am. J. Med.**, v. 79, p. 2531, 1985. Suppl 2 A.

MCKELLAR, P. P. Treatment of community acquired pneumonia. **Am J Crit Care**, v. 11, p. 280, 2002.

MCNEILL H. E. Biting back at poor oral hygiene. Intensive **Crit. Care Nurs.** V. 16, p. 367372, 2000.

MEDURI, G. U. Diagnosis of ventilator associated pneumonia. **Infect. Dis. Clin. North Am.**, Philadelphia, v. 7, n. 2, p. 295-329, jun 1993.

MEGRAN, D.; W.; CHOW, A. W. Bacterial aspiration and anaerobic pleuropulmonary infections. In: SANDE, M. A.; HUDSON, L. D.; ROOT, R. K. (eds). **Respiratory infections.** New York: Churchill Livingstone; 1986. P. 269-92.

MEURMAN, J. H. et al. Hospital mouth-cleaning aids may cause dental erosion. **Spec. Care Dentist**, v. 16, n. 6, p. 247-50, 1996.

MEURMAN, J. H.; TEN CATE, J. M. Pathogenesis and modifying factors of dental erosion. **Eur. J. Sci.**, v. 104, n. , p. 199-206, 1996.

MONTENEGRO, F. L. B. Update on odontogeriatrics. **Vioral (MSD)**, v. 3, n. 8, p. 5, mai./ago. 2003.

MOORE, J. Assesment of nurse-administered oral hygiene. **Nurs. Times,** v. 91, n. 9, p. 40-1, Marc.1995.

MORAIS, T. M. N. et al. The importance of dental care for patients in intensive care units. **Rev. Bras. Ter. Intensiva**. v. 18, n. 4, p. 412-417, 2006.

MORAIS, T. M. N.; SILVA, A.; KNOBEL, E.; AVI A. L. R. O.; LIA R. C. C. **Patients in the Intensive Care Unit: Joint Action by Doctors and Dental Surgeons.** In: Serrano Jr CV; Oliveira MCM; Lotufo RFM; Moraes RGB; Morais TMN. (Cardiology and Dentistry. An integrated vision. 1 ed. São Paulo: Editora Santos, v. 1, p. 249-270, 2007.

MUNRO, C. L. et al. Oral health on VAP (abstract). **Am. J. Crit. Care**, v. 11, p. 280, 2002.

NASCIMENTO, D. F. F.; SILVA, A. M.; MARCHINI, L. **The role of oral bacteria in systemic diseases**. 2005. In press.

NELSON S., LAUGHON B. E.; SUMMER W. R. et al. Characterisation of the pulmonary inflammatory response to an anaerobic bacterial challenge. **Am. Rev. Respir. Dis.**, 133, p. 212-217, 1986.

PEARSON, L. S. A comparison of the ability of foam swabs and toothbrushes to remove dental plaque: implications for nursing practice. **J. Adv. Nurs**., v. 23, p. 62-69, 1996.

PELTOLA P., VEHKALAHTI M. M.; WUOLIJOKI-SAARISTO, K. Oral health and treatment needs of the long-term hospitalised elderly. **The Gerontology Association**, n. 21, p. 93-99, June 2004.

POTTER, P. A.; PERRY, A. G. **Fundamentals of Nursing.** Rio de Janeiro: Guanabara Koogan, 4. ed, v. 1 e 2, p. 518-539, 1999...

PUGIN, R. et al. Oropharyngeal Decontamination Decreases Incidence of Ventilator- Associated Pneumonia: A Randomised, Placebo-Controlled, Double-Blind Clinical Trial. **Jama**, v. 265, n. 20, p. 2704-2710, May. 1991.

PUPULIM, J. S. L.; SAWADA, N. O. Nursing care and the invasion of patient privacy: an ethical-moral issue. **Rev. Latino-Am. Enfermagem**, v.10, n. 3, p. 433-38, mai./jun. 2002.

PURICELLI, E; WELLS, H. The Hospital Face of Dentistry. **Rev. ABO Nac.**, v. 4, n. 1, feb./mar. 1996.

RANSIER, A et al. A combined analysis of a toothbrush, foam brush, and a chlorhexidine- soaked foam brush in maintaining oral hygiene. **Cancer Nurs.,** v. 18, n. 5, p. 393-6, 1995.

RELLO J. et al. Oral care practices in intensive care units: a survey of 59 European ICUs. **Intensive Care Med.,** v. 33, n. 6. p.1066-70, Jun. 2007.

RENTON-HARPER, P. et al. A comparison of chlorexidine, cetylpyridinium chloride, triclosan and C31G mouthrinse products for plaque inhibition. **J. Periodontol.**, Chicago, v. 67, n. 5, p. 486-489, May1996.

REYNOLDS, M. W.. Education for geriatric oral health promotion. **Spec. Care Dent.,** v.17, n. 1, p. 33-36, Ja./Feb.1997.

REZENDE, T. O. **Análise dos cuidados bucais realizadas pela equipe de enfermagem em pacientes idosos hospitalizados na cidade de Uberlândia, Minas Gerais.** São Paulo, 2005. 177f. Monograph (Specialisation in Odontogeriatrics)-Dentistry Subdivision, Brazilian Association of Dental Education (ABENO).

ROSENTHAL, S.; TAGER, I. B. Prevalence of gram-negative rods in the normal pharyngeal flora. Ann Intern Med. v. 83, n. 3, p. 355-357, Sep.1975.

ROTH P. T.; CREASON N. S. Nurse administered oral hygiene: is there a scientific basis? **J. Adv. Nurs.**, v. 11, n. 3, p. 323-31, May 1986.

SAFAR, P.; CAROLINE, N. Acute respiratory failure. In: SCHWARTZ, G.R. **Emergências médicas**. Rio de Janeiro: Interamericana, 1982. Chap. 3, p. 50-97.

SAFDAR, N.; CRNICH, C. J.; MAKI, D. G. The pathogenesis of ventilatorassociated pneumonia: its relevance to developing effective strategies for prevention. **Respir. Care,** v. 50, n. 6, p. 725-39, 2005.

SCANNAPIECO FA, STEWART EM, MYLOTTE JM. Colonisation of dental plaque by respiratory pathogens in medical intensive care patients. **Crit. Care Med.** v. 20, n. 6, p. 740745, 1992.

SCANNAPIECO, F. A.; PAPANDONATOS, G. D.; DUNFORD, R. G. Associations between oral conditions and respiratory disease in a national sample survey population. **Ann. Periodontol.**, v. 3, p. 251-256, 1998.

SECCO, L. G.; PEREIRA, M. L. T. Dental trainers: teaching professionalisation and political-structural challenges. **Ciênc. Saúde Coletiva**. v. 9, n. 1, p. 113-20, 2004.

SEGRETTI, J. Nosocomial infections and secondary infections in sepsis. **Crit. Care Clin.**, v. 5, p. 177-189, 1989.

SILVA A. F. M.; MORAES, C. P. Estudo dos métodos de higiene bucal aplicados em pacientes internados na UTI. 2005. SIMIONATO, M. R. L. **Oral microbiology**. Available at: <http://icb.usb.br/%7Ebmm/materiais/Apostila%20BMM%200560%20-%20Noturno.pdf> Accessed on: 10 July 2006.

SIMIONATO, M. R. L. Oral microbiology. Available at: HTTP://icb.usp.br%7Ebmm/materiais/Apostila%20BMM%200560%20Noturno.pdf Accessed on: 10 July 2006.

SOUZA, V. M. S.; PAGANI, C.; JORGE, A. L. C. Odontogeriatria: suggestion for a prevention programme. **PRG Pós - Grad Rev. Fac. Odontol.**, São José dos Campos, v. 4, n. 1 jan./abr. 2001.

SPIJKERVET, F. K. L.; et al. Effect of selective elimination of the oral flora on mucosites in irradiated head and neck cancer patients. **J. Surg. Oncol.**, v. 46, n. 3, p. 167-73, Mar.1991.

STEELE, J. G. et al. How do age and tooth loss affect oral health and quality of life? A study comparing two national samples. Community Dent oral epidemiol. **Community Det. Oral Epidemiol.**, v.32, n.2, p.107-114, Apr. 2004. Available at: <www.nature.com/cgi-taf/dynapage.taf?file=/bdj/journal/v197/n7/full/4811715a.html> Accessed on: 09/10/2004.

STIEFEL, K. A. et al. Improving oral hygiene for the seriously ill patient: implementing research-based practice. **Medsurg. Nurs.**, v. 9, n.1, 40-3, 46, Feb. 2000.

STOUTENBEEK, C. P.; HENDRIK, H. K. F.; MIRANDA, D. R. The effect of oropharygeal decontamination using topical nonabsorbable antibiotics on the incidence of nosocomial respiratory tract infections in multiple trauma patients. **J. Trauma,** v. 27, p. 357-364, 1987.

TIMBY, B. K. **Fundamental concepts and skills in nursing care.** 6. ed. Porto Alegre: Artmed, 2001. p. 961-968.

TOEWS, G. B. Nosocomial pneumonia. **Am. J. Med. Sci**, v. 291, p. 355-367, 1986.

TREOLAR D. M.; STECHMILLER J. K. Use of a clinical assessment tool for orally intubated patients. **Am. J. Crit. Care,** v. 4, n. 5, p. 355-60, 1995.

TURANO J. C.; TURANO L. M. **Fundamentos de prótese total**. 6. ed. São Paulo: Editora Santos, 1998. p. 75-91.

VAN STRYDONCK, D. A. C. et al. Plaque inhibition of two commercially available chlorhexidine mouthrinses. **J. Clin. Periodontol.,** v. 32, n. 3, p. 305-9, Mar. 2005.

VILELA, E. M., MENDES I. J. M. Interdisciplinaridade e Saúde: Estudo Bibliográfico. **Rev. Latino-Am. Enfermagem**, v.11, n. 4, jul./aug., 2003, p.525-531.

WAITZBERG, D. L.; RODRIGUES, J. G.; CORREIA, M. I. T. D. Hospital malnutrition in Brazil. **In: ___. Oral, enteral and parenteral nutrition in clinical practice.** Atheneu, 1998. Chap. 24, p. 385-397.

WALL, R. J. et al. Protocol-driven care in the intensive care unit: a tool for quality. **Critcal Care**. v. 5, p. 283-285, 2001.

WASH, T. S. et al. Evaluation of simple criteria to predict successful weaning from mechanical ventilation in intensive care patients. **British Journal of Anaesthesia**. v. 6, p. 793-799, 2004.

WENZEL, R. P. Hospital-acquired infection. In: BALLOWS A.; HAUSLER, W. J.; HERRMANN, K. I. **Manual of clinical microbiology**. Washington: American Society for Microbiology, 1991. p. 147-50.

WENZEL, R. P. Hospital-acquired pneumonia: overview of the current state of the art prevention and control. **Eur. J. Clin. Microbiol. Infect. Dis.**, v. 8, p. 56-60, 1989.

WHITE, D. J. An alcohol-free therapeutic mouthrinse with cetypyridinium chloride (CPC) - The latest advance in preventive care: Crest Pro-Health Rinse. **Am. J. Dent.**, v. 18 (special issue), p. 3a-8a, 2005.

ZIVIANI, C. H.; CRUZ, F. P. **Possible relationship between inadequate oral hygiene and the appearance of respiratory infections in ICU patients. Belém**. 2006. Monograph (Graduation Course Final Paper) - Federal University of Pará.

APPENDICES

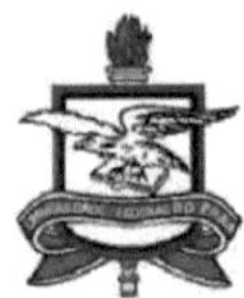

Belém, 23rd May 2007

To the Hospital ________
ATT. Clinical Management
Nursing Coordinator

Dear Dr

I would like to take the liberty of introducing you to Dr Rodolfo José Gomes de Araújo, a dental surgeon from this city and a student on the postgraduate master's course at the Federal University of Pará.

As part of his dissertation, the student has to present a study on the area and, among the various topics chosen, Dr Rodolfo Araújo had to obtain a profile of how oral care is perceived and carried out with patients in Intensive Care Units.

To analyse how the nursing staff (in all its functional segments) perceives and practices oral care for the patients under their responsibility. The research is being proposed by means of questionnaires, which will be applied by the aforementioned Dental Surgeon, in order to avoid calibration errors between different interviewers. The questionnaires have already been tested and are very quick to complete, taking nurses an average of 4.50 minutes to complete.

The interviewees' names will be kept confidential, and they will not be photographed or filmed in any way. The hospital's name will also be preserved in any part of the dissertation work or in scientific articles that we may publish later based on the results obtained.

Despite the physical distance that separates us, I ask for your co-operation in helping him with this work, giving him access to the groups involved in the various work shifts, always with the certainty that his visit will be discreet and as quick as possible so as not to harm anyone.

Thank you in advance for anything you can do to help us in this difficult task of seeking the well-being of hospitalised patients.

Reiterating my best wishes,

Yours sincerely,

Prof Dr Adriano Maia Corrêa
PhD in Periodontics from the University of São Paulo
Adjunct Professor I at the Federal University of Pará
Professor at the Pará Higher Education Centre

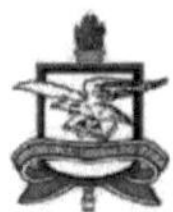

FEDERAL PUBLIC SERVICE
FEDERAL UNIVERSITY OF PARÁ POSTGRADUATE COURSE IN DENTISTRY - MASTER'S LEVEL INFORMED CONSENT FORM

I am being invited to take part in a study on the perceptions and oral care provided by nursing staff in intensive care units, which is being carried out by a master's degree student at the Federal University of Pará in public and private healthcare institutions in the city of Belém.

In order for me to decide whether or not to take part in the research, I was given the following information:

1. The title of the project is: Analysis of Perceptions and Actions on Oral Care Carried Out by Nursing Teams in Intensive Care Units in the City of Belém.
2. The lead researcher is dental surgeon Rodolfo José Gomes de Araújo, who is studying for a master's degree in dentistry at the Federal University of Pará.
3. The aim of the research is to analyse the opinions and oral hygiene procedures that are being carried out by professionals who are part of nursing teams towards ICU patients.
4. This research is risk-free.
5. Questionnaires with multiple-choice questions will be offered to ICU professionals.
6. The research in question has been approved by the Research Ethics Committee of the Federal University of Pará, as shown in the annex.
7. No one is obliged to take part in the research, and anyone can leave the research at any time, as there will be no personal harm from this.
8. There will be no charge for taking part in the research, nor will there be any form of payment for taking part.
9. The great benefit of this research for all those who take part is that it will provide greater knowledge about oral hygiene procedures carried out by nurses, technicians and nursing assistants in ICU patients, enabling treatment strategies to improve the quality of life of these patients.
10. Participation in the research is confidential, which means that only the researcher will know about your participation. The names of the interviewees and the institutions visited will not be disclosed. The data used in the research will only be used in this work.

Signature of the Researcher in Charge

FREE AND INFORMED CONSENT

I declare that I have read the above information about the research, that I feel fully informed about its content, as well as its risks and benefits. I also declare that, of my own free will, I agree to take part in the research by co-operating with the collection of material for examination.

Bethlehem, / /

Participant's signature

Prontuário:

Protocol:

DENTISTRY COURSE. Universidade Federal do Pará, Centro de Ciências da Saúde, Programa de Pós- Graduação-Nível Mestrado - Rua Augusto Corrêa, 01 CEP 66075-110 - Caixa postal 479 PABX +55 91 32017000 - Belém - Pará - Brasil e-mail: rjga@ufpa.br

RESEARCH ETHICS COMMITTEE CEP-CCS/UFPA. Universidade Federal do Pará - Complexo de Aulas/CCS - Sala 14 - Campus Universitário do Guamá, 66075-110 - Belém, Pará, Tel.: (91) 3201-8028, e-mail: cepccs@ufpa.br

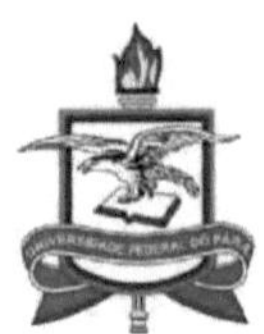

FEDERAL UNIVERSITY OF PARÁ
MASTER'S PROGRAMME IN DENTISTRY

RESEARCHER RESPONSIBLE: RODOLFO ARAÚJO

Questionnaire for nursing staff N^B _________

01- Which professional category do you work in?

( ) Nurse ( ) Nursing technician ( ) Nursing assistant

02- Age: ______ years

03- Sex: ( ) Female ( ) Male

04- Monthly income:

( ) Up to 2 minimum wages (R$ 520.00) ( ) Up to R$ 1,000.00
( ) Between R$1,000.00 and R$2,000.00 ( ) Above R$ 2,000.00

05- In which type(s) of establishment(s) do you work?

( ) Private hospital ( ) Public hospital
( ) Private clinics ( ) Basic health units
( ) Own home care service ( ) Other _________

06- Time spent training in the area:

( ) less than 1 year ( ) between 1-5 years
( ) more than 5 years ( ) more than 10 years

07- How often do you take refresher courses (seminars, congresses, lectures...)?

( ) I do it often (2 or more times/year)
( ) I do it every year
( ) I don't do it because of the high cost of courses
( ) I don't do it because I don't see how it applies to everyday life

08- Do you work in a multi/interdisciplinary team?

( ) Yes ( ) No

If so, does this group have a dental surgeon as a permanent member?

( ) Yes ( ) No

09- Do you consider it necessary to have a dental surgeon on the team, who could help you in cases where dentistry is involved?

( ) Yes ( ) No

10- Did you know that an infection in the mouth can damage the health of the rest of your body?

( ) Yes ( ) No

11- Do you believe that sanitising your mouth is important during your hospital stay?

( ) Yes ( ) No

12- With regard to the oral care you provide and/or advise your patients on, correlate the column on the left with the one on the right:

(A) Frequent use
(B) Occasional use
(C) No use

( ) Examination of the oral cavity
( ) Normal tooth brushing
( ) Aspiration of the tube in the nasal and oral cavity mouth
( ) Use of a bedside brushing bowl
( ) Mouthwash - What brand do you use?
( ) Hygienisation with gauze on a stick and antiseptic
What brand is used? ______________________
( ) Hygienising dentures (dentures, bridges...)
( ) Discontinuing the use of prostheses (dentures, bridges...)

13- With regard to the prostheses that patients wear, what recommendations are followed in the ICU?

PATIENT CONDITIONS	DO NOT USE	USE
Intubated patients		
Patients after removal of intubation		
Patients with an oro-gastric tube		
Patients with naso-gastric or enteral tubes		
Conscious patients		
Patients with mucosal lesions		

14- Which of the following subjects do you know and are you able to advise your patient on?

( ) Tooth brushing techniques
( ) Normal aspects of the mouth
( ) Most common diseases of the oral cavity (dental caries, gingivitis, periodontitis and others)
( ) Hygienisation of dentures and discontinuation of use
( ) Sanitising mucous membranes
( ) Tongue cleaning

14- Tick the resources used for oral hygiene that you know and/or use in your work environment for your patients:

HYGIENE FEATURE	I DON'T KNOW	I KNOW	I USE
Toothbrush			
Toothpaste			
Dental floss			
Interdental brush			
Tongue cleaner			
Electric brush			
Denture brush			
Mouthwash			
Fluoride solutions			
Floss threader			
Artificial saliva			
Gel/paste for fixing dentures			
Wooden toothpick			

16- Do you advise your patients to see a dentist periodically for an oral cavity examination and oral cancer prevention?

( ) Yes ( ) No

17- Did you receive specific training in oral hygiene during your training?

( ) Yes ( ) No

If so, how would you classify them?

( ) Sufficient to take care of patients' oral problems
( ) Insufficient to take care of patients' oral problems

18- Would you like to learn more about oral health and apply this knowledge to your patients?

( ) Yes ( ) No

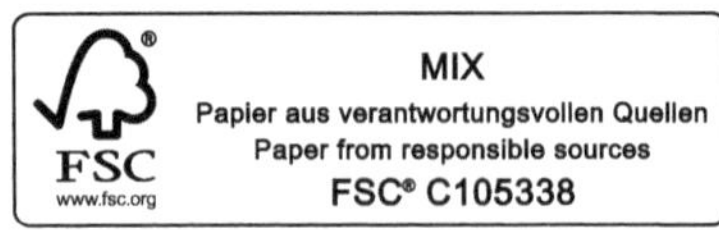

Printed by Books on Demand GmbH, Norderstedt / Germany